Effective *Peer* Review

THIRD EDITION

The Complete Guide
to Physician Performance
Improvement

Robert J. Marder, MD

Effective Peer Review: The Complete Guide to Physician Performance Improvement, Third Edition is published by HCPro, Inc.

Copyright © 2013 HCPro, Inc.

All rights reserved. Printed in the United States of America.   5 4 3 2 1

ISBN: 978-1-60146-965-6

No part of this publication may be reproduced, in any form or by any means, without prior written consent of HCPro, Inc., or the Copyright Clearance Center (978-750-8400). Please notify us immediately if you have received an unauthorized copy.

HCPro, Inc., provides information resources for the healthcare industry.

HCPro, Inc., is not affiliated in any way with The Joint Commission, which owns the JCAHO and Joint Commission trademarks.

Robert J. Marder, MD, Author
Karen Kondilis, Editor
Jim DeWolf, Editorial Director
Shane Katz, Art Director; Cover Designer
Mike Mirabello, Graphic Artist
Matt Sharpe, Production Supervisor
Jean St. Pierre, Vice President of Operations and Customer Relations

Advice given is general. Readers should consult professional counsel for specific legal, ethical, or clinical questions.

Arrangements can be made for quantity discounts. For more information, contact:

HCPro, Inc.
75 Sylvan Street, Suite A-101
Danvers, MA 01923
Telephone: 800-650-6787 or 781-639-1872
Fax: 800-639-8511
Email: *customerservice@hcpro.com*

Visit HCPro online at *www.hcpro.com* and *www.hcmarketplace.com*

05/2013
22035

Contents

About the Author ix
Dedication xi
Introduction xiii

Chapter 1: Peer Review: Why Do We Need to Evaluate Physician Competence? 1

What Peer Review Is 2

What Peer Review Is Not 4

Who Is a Peer? 7

Impartiality and Conflicts of Interest 8

Sham Peer Reviews 10

The Duty to Perform Effective Peer Review 10

Should Physicians Be Paid to Perform Peer Reviews? 13

Physician Leader–Driven Peer Review: A Medical Staff Leader's View 13

Chapter 2: From Punitive to Positive: Creating a Performance Improvement Culture for Peer Review 17

How Can Culture Change? 18

Values of a Performance Improvement–Focused Peer Review Culture 19

Peer Review and the Just Culture 32

CONTENTS

Chapter 3: Legal Considerations: Impact of Regulations and Liability on Peer Review **35**

Redefining Peer Review: OPPE, FPPE, and the Core Competencies 35

How the Standards Apply 38

Peer Review Protection Laws 41

Affirmative Duty to Keep Information Confidential 44

Fair Hearings 45

The National Practitioner Data Bank 45

Negligent Peer Review 47

Chapter 4: Peer Review Structures: The Impact of Multi-Specialty Peer Review **49**

Peer Review Structures: Three Primary Functions 50

Goals for Peer Review Structure Design 52

Basic Peer Review Models 53

Who Should Oversee Peer Review? 59

Selecting the Right Model 59

Multidisciplinary Membership and Participation in Peer Review 61

Physician Behavior: Who Should Handle It? 61

Chapter 5: Measuring Physician Performance: What to Measure and How to Do It Fairly **63**

What Is a Physician Performance Indicator? 63

Indicator Validity: Selecting Physician-Driven Measures 64

What Are You Required to Measure? 64

What to Measure: Structure, Process, and Outcome 65

How to Measure Physicians Fairly: Review, Rate, and Rule Indicators 68

Understanding and Improving Risk-Adjusted Data 76

Using Perception Data to Evaluate Physician Performance 77

Case Study: Selecting the Right Indicator 80

CONTENTS

Chapter 6: Case Review: Reducing Bias and Improving Reviewer Efficiency and Effectiveness 83

    Standardizing the Case Review Process 83

    Case Identification and Screening 84

    Physician Reviewer Assignment 88

    Physician Review and Initial Case Rating 89

    Initial Committee Review and Physician Input 92

    Committee Decision and Improvement Opportunity Identification 95

    Communication of Findings and Follow-Up Accountability 96

    Case Rating Systems 97

    Case Review and the Electronic Age 99

    Case Study: Who Is in Charge? 100

Chapter 7: Selecting Physician-Driven Measures for OPPE: Understanding and Applying the Six Core Competencies 105

    ACGME, ABMS, and The Joint Commission: Where Did the Core Competencies Come From and How Are They Used? 106

    Alternative Frameworks to the Core Competencies 108

    Using the Competency Statement and Expectations to Drive Physician Performance Measures 110

    Applying the Core Competencies to OPPE 116

Chapter 8: Physician Data Attribution: Making OPPE Data Meaningful to Individual Physicians 119

    Using Imprecise Data for OPPE 120

    Attribution and Case Review 122

    Improving Attribution for Process Measures 123

    Outcome Measure Attribution in a Multiple Provider World 125

    Attribution and Patient Satisfaction Data 126

    Case Study: Engaging the Medical Staff in Attribution 128

CONTENTS

Chapter 9: Evaluating OPPE Data: Using Benchmarks and Targets for FPPE and the Pursuit of Excellence 129

Understanding Normative Data 130

Interpreting OPPE Data for a Time Interval 132

How to Set Indicator Targets 134

Targets for Indicator Types 137

Interpreting OPPE Data for Trends 140

Chapter 10: From OPPE to FPPE: Creating Accountability for Physician Performance Improvement 143

Accountability for FPPE Initiation, Monitoring, and Follow-Up 144

Designing an Effective FPPE Plan 146

Getting Physician Buy-In for Improvement Opportunities and FPPE 147

What Happens if FPPE Fails? 149

FPPE for New Members and Privileges: Why Is It Different? 150

Case Study: Initiating an FPPE for Mortality Data 151

Chapter 11: OPPE Profiles and Physician Performance Feedback: Practical Principles for Competency Report Design and Distribution 157

OPPE Profile and Physician Performance Feedback Report: What Is the Difference? 157

Design the Report 158

Define the Principles: 10 Questions to Guide Your Design 159

Create a Format That Reflects the Design Principles 163

Prepare and Distribute Competency Data Reports 172

Develop the Infrastructure and Support Materials 172

Pilot-Test Your Design 176

Create a Policy for Physician Competency Reports 179

CONTENTS

Chapter 12: External Peer Review in a Physician Improvement Culture ... 183

- EPR Uses ... 183
- The EPR Policy ... 184
- What Circumstances Typically Require EPR? ... 184
- Who Determines When EPR Is Needed? ... 186
- Who Will Select the Reviewer? ... 188
- How Will the Cases Be Selected? ... 188
- Who Will Review the EPR Report Findings? ... 190
- How Will the Results Be Used? ... 191
- Beyond Case-Based EPR: Physician Assessment Programs ... 191

Chapter 13: Reporting Peer Review: What Does the Board Need to Know? ... 193

- Contemporary Board Accountabilities for Hospital Quality ... 193
- What Keeps the Board Awake at Night? ... 194
- Filling in the Knowledge Gap: Helping Boards Understand Physician Competency Measurement ... 195
- What Data Should the Board Get? ... 196

Chapter 14: Running an Effective Peer Review Committee Meeting ... 203

- Elements of an Effective Meeting ... 204
- Role of the Committee Chair ... 205
- Responsibilities of Committee Members in Meeting Preparation and Management ... 206
- Practical Tips for Managing Committee Discussion to Avoid Wasting Physician Time ... 207

Chapter 15: Beyond the Hospital Walls: Peer Review in Ambulatory Care and ACOs ... 211

- Why Would You Want to Do Peer Review in a Nonhospital Setting? ... 211
- Can You Do Peer Review in the Nonhospital Setting? ... 213
- What Data Can You Obtain From the Hospital and What Are You Willing to Share? ... 213
- Peer Review Outside the Hospital: How Should You Organize It? ... 215
- Peer Review Outside the Hospital: What Can You Measure? ... 220

CONTENTS

Chapter 16: Creating Effective Peer Review Policies and Procedures 225

What Do Your Policies and Procedures Need to Cover? 225

Redesigning Your Peer Review Program: A Step-by-Step Guide 227

Should You Do This Yourself or Get Some Help? 229

About the Author

Robert J. Marder, MD, is president of Robert J. Marder Consulting, LLC. Dr. Marder brings more than 30 years of healthcare leadership, management, and consulting experience to his work with physicians, hospitals, and healthcare organizations nationwide. A highly respected speaker, consultant, and author, he has assisted hundreds of hospital medical staffs evaluate and improve their approach to peer review and physician performance measurement.

Marder is the former vice president of The Greeley Company, a division of HCPro, Inc., in Danvers, Mass., and served as practice director for medical staff consulting. In this role, for over 12 years he has consulted with hospitals and healthcare systems throughout the country in the areas of hospital and medical staff performance improvement, peer review, patient safety, medical staff development, and case management.

He previously served as vice president for medical affairs at Holy Cross Hospital in Chicago and as medical director for quality management and assistant vice president for quality management at Rush Presbyterian-St. Luke's Medical Center in Chicago.

Marder began his full-time involvement in performance improvement in 1988 as the national project director for clinical indicator development and use at the Joint Commission on Accreditation of Healthcare Organizations (JCAHO) in Oak Brook Terrace, Ill. During his three years there, he managed five expert national task forces developing indicators for the JCAHO Agenda for Change and conducted extensive training workshops in the use of performance measures in quality improvement.

Marder is a board-certified pathologist and former assistant director of laboratories and director of the clinical immunology laboratory at Chicago-based Northwestern Memorial Hospital. He received his undergraduate degree from the University of Illinois-Champaign and his medical degree from Rush Medical College.

For more information, visit *www.robertjmarderconsulting.com*.

Dedication

This book is dedicated to physicians on medical staffs across the country who perform this difficult task, without any or minimal compensation, to fulfill their professional responsibility to improve the profession's standards and performance for the good of our patients and communities.

I would like to thank Dr. Mary Hoppa from The Greeley Company for her assistance in reviewing the regulatory standards chapter and for her consulting work with me in peer review redesign over the past six years. I would also like to acknowledge the consultants from The Greeley Company who served as co-authors for the previous editions of this book. In particular, I want to thank Dr. Richard Sheff, whose work in this area formed the basis for the approach used to create a performance improvement focused peer review.

Finally, I would like to dedicate this book to my wonderful wife of 36 years, Susanne, whose demonstration of grace beyond anything I ever deserved has been a continuous inspiration to me.

Introduction

In 1916, E.A. Codman, a founder of the American College of Surgeons and an early crusader for quality improvement, stated the need for peer review and a quality program for healthcare delivered at the hospital level. Today, peer review—the practice of physicians reviewing the work of other physicians—is considered a crucial element of ensuring that patients are provided with quality medical care.

There is no question that peer review has evolved from the professional obligation physicians have long felt to ensure that safe care was being provided in their community. Today, accreditors, federal and state laws, and medical staff bylaws require that hospitals have a process by which to review physician performance. In addition, the legal doctrine of corporate negligence imposes a duty on hospitals to select and maintain competent staff. Finally, as government and commercial payers' interest in the quality of patient care has expanded beyond the acute care setting, evaluating physician care will be a necessary element of that process.

The methods of peer review have also evolved. It is no longer limited to physicians reviewing individual charts with poor clinical outcomes or conducting a subjective evaluation at the bi-annual reappointment evaluation. Following the lead of other high risk industries, such as aviation and nuclear power, peer review is being challenged to become a data driven, ongoing performance improvement process.

As with the previous two editions, this book discusses how to create an effective peer review program based on these contemporary concepts. Recognizing that this process will vary depending on each hospital's and each medical staff's culture, resources, and circumstances, this book is designed to help you in two ways. First, it provides a background and framework to help the reader understand how peer review can be a positive force for physician improvement. Second, it provides practical, tested strategies based on working with medical staffs across the country over the past 12 years to make that change a reality.

So why have we updated this book? In the first edition, this broader approach to peer review was predominately considered a best practice rather than a regulatory requirement. By the second edition,

INTRODUCTION

regulations had caught up with best practice (the changes in 2007 Joint Commission medical staff standards) so the book's goal was to incorporate the regulatory needs into the best practices. In addition, I was also the lead author on two other related books published by HCPro, *Measuring Physician Competency* and *Peer Review Best Practices: Case Studies and Lessons Learned,* designed to fill in some of the gaps related to the implementation of these concepts.

This third edition is designed to combine all three related books into a single volume that provides a comprehensive view of peer review. While recognizing the regulatory needs for peer review, the overriding theme of this edition is how to keep the focus of peer review on physician improvement and the pursuit of excellence. Today, most medical staffs have figured out how to meet the minimal regulatory requirements. However, many still struggle with how to effectively improve physician care in a non-punitive culture; despite their best intentions, their peer review program is still perceived as punitive.

While this edition certainly builds on the previous ones, most of the chapters of this edition have been substantially revised to reflect what has been learned by experience in the past five years. This edition also addresses the evolving need for peer review in non-hospital settings. As physicians are challenged with new organizational structures for delivering patient care, how physician care will be evaluated and improved and who will be accountable for that function will be critical to the success of these new ventures.

Thus, I hope that this book can assist physicians, whether they are in a hospital medical staff, primary care group, multi-specialty group practice, or accountable care organization, as they perform this role in a manner that maintains their professional obligation to their patients with the collegiality and dignity they deserve.

Peer Review: Why Do We Need to Evaluate Physician Competence?

"The thing that hath been, it is that which shall be; and that which is done is that which shall be done: and there is no new thing under the sun."

Ecclesiastes 1:9 (KJV).

Peer review is not new. As a profession, physicians have long shown the desire to evaluate and improve the care they provide to their patients. They have done this, and still do it, because of the very reason physicians choose this profession: to help make people well to the best of the physician's knowledge and ability.

However, in contrast to the verse from Ecclesiastes, some things have changed. In the past, physician performance evaluation was considered the sacred province of the medical staff, not to be shared with the rest of the world. Patients never considered asking a physician for data regarding the outcomes of care. Even accreditation bodies only looked to be sure a process was in place with the medical staff to conduct this performance function, but did not evaluate the actual results.

Today is a different story. Although the concept of sharing data publicly goes back to Ernest Codman in the late 1800s, in the past decade, through the combination of growing public interest and advances in information technology, healthcare data that was once secret is now transparent. Data that once focused on the hospital level is increasingly becoming physician-specific and available to the public; and there is no indication of any reversal of this trend.

What about the evaluation of that data by other physicians? Peer review is still protected from disclosure in the vast majority of states. However, since the raw data is becoming more available, the public may draw its own conclusions without the benefit of the more in-depth understanding of underlying factors that might explain the data.

So if the public will have the data, why should physicians even bother to perform peer review? First, accrediting bodies have been increasing their scrutiny of the peer review process to justify its effectiveness and eventually its existence. Peer review is a privilege that society, through the accreditation process, has granted physicians. It is not a right.

Beyond the need to meet regulatory requirements, a compelling reason for renewed engagement by physicians is that when peer review is done well, it provides the opportunity for the medical profession to get ahead of the curve with respect to data transparency. If physicians can identify and address the issues driving physician performance early on, then the subsequent data available to the public will be substantially better. The overall goal of this book is to assist physician leaders to help make the transition from regulatory-driven to performance improvement–driven peer review.

What Peer Review Is

Peer review is the evaluation of an individual physician's professional performance by other physicians, the identification of opportunities to improve physician care, and a way to help physicians achieve those improvements. Traditionally, this process has been executed by physician peers reviewing charts of individual cases that were selected for review based on adverse outcomes criteria, such as complications or mortality.

Psychologist Abraham Maslow said, "If the only tool you have is a hammer, everything looks like a nail." Today, medical staffs have more tools to evaluate a physician's performance than just the "hammer" of individual chart review. Such tools include rate and rule indicators, which will be discussed in later chapters. Most medical staffs are in the process of adding these tools to their belts.

Moreover, there is growing recognition that there are more dimensions to physician performance than just the technical quality of care provided. This is reflected in The Joint Commission's adoption of the Accreditation Council for Graduate Medical Education's (ACGME) and the American Board of Medical Specialties' (ABMS) six core competencies, which will be discussed in Chapter 7. The six core competencies are:

- Patient care
- Medical knowledge
- Interpersonal skills
- Professionalism

PEER REVIEW: WHY DO WE NEED TO EVALUATE PHYSICIAN COMPETENCE?

- Systems-based practice

- Practiced-based learning

As a result, this book suggests a more contemporary definition of peer review:

Peer review is the evaluation of all dimensions of current competency of individual physicians using all appropriate and relevant sources of performance data available.

Peer review is required by The Joint Commission, the American Osteopathic Association Healthcare Facilities Accreditation Program, and Det Norske Veritas (DNV) hospital-accreditation standards, federal laws such as those governing Medicare and Medicaid programs, state laws, and each hospital's own bylaws. As will be discussed in Chapter 15, peer review is also becoming an important element in ambulatory care and accountable care organization quality programs.

The physician peer review process has two components. The first is the initial review of a physician's qualifications to determine whether that physician may be granted the privilege to perform specific procedures or treat specific diseases. Once the privilege is granted, the organization may evaluate the initial use of the privilege by the physician in its own setting for a focused period of time (e.g., three months). This peer evaluation, now termed focused professional practice evaluation (FPPE), is typically performed by the hospital credentialing committee and occurs at the physician's initial appointment or when a new privilege is requested. This component of peer review is not the subject of this book.

The second component of peer review is the ongoing monitoring of a physician's use of those privileges for patient care. There are two phases of this ongoing review. The first phase, termed ongoing professional practice evaluation (OPPE), involves the systematic collection and review of individual physician data to identify potential improvement opportunities. The second phase, also termed FPPE, which follows OPPE, involves either more in-depth data collection or working with the physician to improve and then monitor the results. The results of both OPPE, and any related FPPE, are then used for the decision every two years to either renew or restrict a physician's privileges or membership. This component of peer review is the primary focus of this book. However, as discussed in Chapter 2, peer review is much more useful if it is done with the goal of physician improvement and not just as a mechanism for reappointment.

CHAPTER 1

What Peer Review Is Not

As approaches to peer review have evolved, two methods for understanding and improving patient care, mortality and morbidity (M&M) conferences and root cause analysis (RCA), are sometimes confused with peer review. Although these improvement activities may look at similar events, it is critical to recognize the difference between these methods and official peer review and to keep them as separate functions to ensure that peer review is conducted consistently and fairly.

How does peer review differ from an M&M conference? While the M&M conference can be a valuable component of a medical staff's overall strategy to improve patient care, it needs to be separated from formal peer review because it violates two main principles of peer review:

1. The application of clear conflict-of-interest standards. During an M&M conference, the physician under discussion is present and often actively participates.

2. The variability of the participants that can affect the due process required for peer review. Also, since an M&M is designed as a "y'all come" process, there will be inherent variability in the composition of the group from meeting to meeting.

Because of these issues, when peer review is done through an M&M model, medical staffs often report difficulties in arriving at fair decisions and defining effective improvements. Therefore, the M&M conference should be solely an educational session. In this context, it can be a collegial open discussion of clinical cases or situations without the burden of making final determinations that will end up in a physician's quality file. This discussion can also involve nonphysician healthcare professionals with an interest in the clinical case. There should be a connection between the peer review process and the M&M conference in two ways:

1. The conference is used as a source of case identification for peer review.

2. Cases from peer review may be later discussed at M&M for educational purposes.

How does peer review differ from RCA? An RCA is a systems analysis required after significant or sentinel events have occurred, such as a wrong site surgery. It is a multidisciplinary effort to identify the causal factors that lead to a variation in performance. As such, RCAs focus primarily on systems and processes, not on individual performance. For example, in a wrong site surgery, an RCA asks the question, "How did our systems and processes fail that we allowed a physician to operate on the wrong site?" Although

PEER REVIEW: WHY DO WE NEED TO EVALUATE PHYSICIAN COMPETENCE?

an RCA looks at human factors most directly associated with the sentinel event, it does not deal with the individual performance of physicians or clinical staff. For the clinical staff, the human resource function would address those issues. For the medical staff, this would be handled by peer review.

Unfortunately, when the medical staff peer review program is ineffective, the multidisciplinary RCA team may be tempted to assume the task of evaluating individual physician performance. The best way to fix this problem is to address its root cause—that is, to strengthen your medical staff peer review process.

13 ANGRY MEN?

Some of the most dramatic movie scenes involve a jury deliberating the fate of a defendant. In fact, the 1957 film *12 Angry Men* was set almost entirely in the jury room. But what if the screenwriter had decided to place the defendant in the jury room and allowed him to comment while the jury argued about the case and determined his fate? You would think that something is terribly wrong with the script.

I pose this scenario because I recently received the following question regarding how to handle a potential conflict of interest during a peer review evaluation:

If a case comes before the peer review committee to discuss and assign a rating, and the case involves a member of the peer review committee, does that member:

1. *Remain in the room to discuss the details of the case?*

2. *Get asked to leave the room when it is time to assign a rating?*

3. *Take part in the entire process, including discussion and rating?*

The best answer is "None of the above." Any practitioner, not just a member of the committee, should not be present during either the discussion or the rating of his or her case. This would be akin to a defendant sitting in a jury room. And yet, The Greeley Company consultants witness this occurrence in many peer review committees. Why do some medical staffs consider having a practitioner present at his or her own case a reasonable approach, but any layperson would be surprised—if not aghast—with this script?

This misconception most likely has its roots in the evolution of peer review, which started as morbidity and mortality (M&M) conferences. During these conferences, the basis for learning required the practitioner to be present so that he or she could explain the case and receive feedback. But M&M conferences are no substitute for peer review. Peer review committees must eliminate, or at least minimize, conflicts of interest through clear policies that are

Effective Peer Review, Third Edition

13 ANGRY MEN? (CONT.)

always adhered to even if they seem inconvenient or not collegial because the practitioner happens to be a committee member.

How should committee members respond when a fellow member's performance is under review? The first step is to inform the practitioner in advance when the case will be discussed so he or she is not caught off-guard and embarrassed. This is best done by the committee chair (rather than by support staff) out of courtesy and respect. The chair should also remind the member of the committee's policy that requires any members who are under review to be absent from the decision. During that discussion, the chair should also ask whether it would be more convenient for the member if the committee discussed the case toward the beginning or end of the meeting, so the member can leave.

The peer review committee should approach cases involving members the same as it would for nonmembers. If your policy states that the peer review committee will write a letter to a practitioner under review asking for an explanation of the case, the same approach should be used for the member. When the committee discusses the response, again, the member cannot be present.

By the way, if your policy does allow for a practitioner to attend the meeting to provide a response, then the policy should limit the practitioner (or the member) to respond only to the committee's questions; the committee should ask the individual to leave during its discussion of the response.

If your medical staff policies allow practitioners to be involved in the review of their own cases, perhaps it is time to re-write that script. One of the most important ways the peer review committee can maintain the credibility of the peer review process is to effectively manage conflicts of interest.

Editor's note: This article was originally published in Medical Staff Leader Insider, *May 6, 2009.*

PEER REVIEW: WHY DO WE NEED TO EVALUATE PHYSICIAN COMPETENCE?

Who Is a Peer?

Traditionally, a peer has been defined as an individual in the same specialty. However, as inpatient medical practice has become more complex, with multiple specialties involved in patient care, numerous handoffs made among practitioners, and increased societal demands for a comprehensive framework that defines quality of care, that definition has proved to be too limited to provide effective peer review.

Many medical staffs have adopted this more contemporary definition of a peer:

A peer is an individual practicing in the same profession and who has expertise in the subject matter under evaluation. The level of subject matter expertise required to provide meaningful evaluation of a provider's performance will be based on the area of competency and the nature of the issue or data being evaluated.

This definition implies that, although a peer of a physician must be another physician, he or she does not necessarily have to be board-certified in the same specialty as the physician whose work is being reviewed. If the question is one of general medical care, or if it is related to issues of responsiveness or communication, any unbiased physician—MD or DO—can serve as a peer reviewer. However, if the question requires evaluation of specialty-specific clinical issues, such as the technique of a specialized surgical procedure, the peer reviewer must be trained and competent in that specialty. The impact of this definition on options for selecting an effective peer review structure is discussed in Chapter 4 and reviewer assignment is discussed in Chapter 6.

For example, assume that an interventional cardiologist, Dr. Coeur, performed a cardiac catheterization. The patient began to bleed in the retroperitoneum and became hypotensive and anuric. Dr. Coeur delayed fluid resuscitation and blood transfusion, and as a result, the patient developed acute renal failure. Did the cardiologist provide appropriate care? Although the question involves care provided by an interventional cardiologist, the actual event that required medical care was a textbook example of basic hemorrhagic shock. Therefore, any physician could be considered capable of evaluating the care provided under this set of circumstances.

Consider another example involving the same cardiologist. This time, Dr. Coeur received a report that a patient who is post-catheterization developed a hematoma at the site of puncture, had decreased hemoglobin by one gram, and was now hypotensive. Dr. Coeur decided not to make any changes and ordered only a follow-up hemoglobin for the morning. By morning, the patient had developed acute renal failure in addition to his earlier problems. Again, any competent physician would recognize that Dr. Coeur's failure to provide sufficient fluid resuscitation and transfusion led to the renal failure.

According to Dr. Harvey Wachsman, a former neurosurgeon who specializes in medical malpractice law, "approximately 70% of all malpractice lawsuits involve the type of slip-ups that would be obvious even to a first-year medical student," such as a physician's failure to be present when needed, failure to take an adequate medical history, or failure to perform an adequate examination. In other words, most of the time, the issue is one of general medical care.

However, there are times when the reviewer must have specialized clinical training. For example, assume that Dr. Coeur had placed multiple stents in a patient's coronary arteries and the patient later suffered a myocardial infarction. Although the general question, "Did Dr. Coeur provide appropriate care?", is the same, this time, however, the answer requires a more technical assessment that only another board-certified interventional cardiologist could make.

Impartiality and Conflicts of Interest

Physician peer review should be as objective and impartial as possible. Unfortunately, individual bias can never be completely eliminated from any form of human evaluation, much less in the context of a medical staff where individuals often know each other. However, peer review bias can be reduced in a number of ways that will be discussed in later chapters.

One of the most important means of bias reduction in peer review is the management of conflict of interest. Because physicians are used to more informal means of interacting in the medical staff meetings, they often are not aware of the need to handle conflicts of interest in a manner that would be considered typical ethical practice in our society.

The ethical obligations of any individual to avoid conflicts of interest are recognition and disclosure. It is the responsibility of the deliberating body to determine whether the disclosed conflict is substantial enough to prevent the individual from participating in the deliberations at hand. For example, a physician peer reviewer with a potential conflict of interest, such as being a weekly golf partner of the physician under review, is ethically obligated to disclose it to the rest of the peer review committee. The committee then will determine whether the conflict is substantial enough to preclude the individual from participation in its discussion and decision. There are a few absolute conflicts of interest, such as when the issues in the case directly involve a:

PEER REVIEW: WHY DO WE NEED TO EVALUATE PHYSICIAN COMPETENCE?

- Reviewer

- Committee member

- Spouse

- First-degree relative

Just as judges who have a personal interest in cases must recuse themselves to avoid even the appearance of impropriety, peer reviewers should recuse themselves in such situations.

Most conflict-of-interest situations, however, are not that clear. For example, some people argue that being a partner or a competitor should be considered an absolute conflict. If it were, however, internal peer review on technical quality of care issues would be virtually impossible. Therefore, these types of conflicts are typically handled as potential conflicts that are addressed on a case-by-case basis.

Another quandary is what to do if a committee member was involved in the care after the event under review occurred—perhaps that physician was even the expert consultant who "rescued" the patient. Some might see that situation as a conflict; others might see that physician as being an excellent source of in-depth information.

Three actions are necessary in order to resolve these potential conflicts of interest so that there will be no question that the peer review was conducted in good faith.

1. The medical staff needs a clear, written conflict-of-interest policy and procedure for peer review to provide guidance on how to handle these situations.

2. All physicians who serve on the peer review committee must be scrupulously honest about disclosing potential conflicts; including relevant personal issues (e.g., the physician under peer review is also engaged in a bitter dispute over a house that was purchased from a committee member).

3. The peer review committee itself must adhere to the policy and use its judgment and wisdom when determining whether a particular physician can render a reasonably objective opinion. This judgment may be based both on the physician's reputation for fairness and on the nature and intensity of the conflict. If the committee has doubts, it should always err on the side of safety and either assign a different reviewer or obtain an external review.

CHAPTER 1

Sham Peer Reviews

Another potential peer review impartiality concern is whether an individual peer reviewer or peer review committee as a whole could be seen as acting in retaliation for a physician's whistle-blowing or raising concerns about patient care. Peer reviews that are biased against the physician for retaliatory or other reasons are sometimes called sham peer reviews.

If a physician has his or her privileges restricted as a result of a sham peer review or of a good-faith peer review that looks biased to an outsider, that physician is much more likely to sue. And when plaintiff physicians challenge the peer review process and are able to prove a case of retaliation or malice, they have, in some instances, been awarded millions of dollars in civil damages. It is easy for a plaintiff's attorney to allege bias, even when none exists, so in this situation, appearances do matter. For this reason, hospitals should carefully define how to handle conflict-of-interest situations so they can avoid even the threat of litigation.

The Duty to Perform Effective Peer Review

A physician's duty to perform good-faith peer review is based in two fundamental principles of medical ethics: the principle of beneficence, or the duty to "do the right thing" and the duty to avoid malfeasance, or "do no harm." In the world of medicine, the duty of beneficence means that physicians have a fiduciary responsibility to act in the best interest of their patients. The Illinois Supreme Court described it well, noting that the physician is "learned, skilled and experienced in those subjects about which the … [patient] ordinarily knows little or nothing … Therefore the patient must necessarily place great reliance, faith and confidence in the professional word, advice and acts of the physician … The essence of the fiduciary relationship is that the patient's interests must be paramount." [1]

The duty to do the right thing for the patient includes a duty to improve care continuously, both for a physician's own patients and for the patient population at large. By joining a medical staff, a physician assumes the obligation to all patients to improve the care provided by all physicians on the staff through participation in peer review.

Physicians aren't the only ones with this duty. The hospital's governing board also has the responsibility to ensure the quality of patient care. However, because most governing boards have little or no expertise in medical quality, they have historically delegated the responsibility of monitoring and

PEER REVIEW: WHY DO WE NEED TO EVALUATE PHYSICIAN COMPETENCE?

improving physician performance to the organized medical staff. Thus, physicians are accountable to the governing board for carrying out effective peer review.

The duty to avoid malfeasance relates to the need to do peer review fairly. When peer review incorrectly determines that a physician has provided poor care, it can do harm to that physician, especially if such a label undermines the physician's ability to grow and sustain a practice. Similarly, when a physician's care is correctly identified as inappropriate, not addressing this issue puts future patients at risk. The key to avoid harmful peer review is to follow clear policies and practices that protect the physician under review and invest in information technology and support that provides a realistic picture of the physician's care.

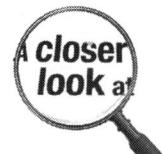

A closer look at: The Question of Compensation

A medical staff professional submitted the following question:

"During our medical staff quality committee meeting, one member commented that committee members should be compensated for their time, especially when serving on committees that involve reviewing material prior to the meeting. I have inquired with my counterparts at other area hospitals. The consensus was that no one is paying committee members. However, the chief of staff, chief elect, department chairs, and vice chairs do receive a stipend.

What are your thoughts on compensating committee members? Should it be all committees or those that require additional time spent outside the actual meeting? Should we pay a flat fee across the board no matter what the physician's specialty, or should the fee reflect the physician's specialty?"

As physicians are more pressed for time to devote to medical staff responsibilities, the burden falls unequally on some more than others. In the past, this was seen as a physician's duty, and compensation was unheard of. Even today, in many medical staff cultures, physicians who are paid for nonclinical work, such as case management or serving as physician advisors or medical directors, are viewed as being "in the pocket" of administration.

So what is the right course? The response to this question should not be construed as either advocating or not advocating physician payment but as a way to begin discussion when approaching the issue with your staff.

There are really four decisions you must make to address this issue:

- Should you pay?

Effective Peer Review, Third Edition

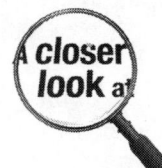

A closer look at: The Question of Compensation (cont.)

- Who should get paid?

- Who should pay?

- How much should you pay?

Should you pay? There is nothing illegal about doing so as long as you are in bounds for the last question of how much to pay. The real issue is what your medical staff members think about physicians getting paid. If your medical staff would react negatively, you need to either work to change that culture or abandon the issue. It's best to discuss this question with your medical executive committee, not with the committee that potentially would be paid.

Who should get paid? Most medical staffs focus on those who go above and beyond rather than on those who just show up at a meeting. Attendance at a committee is part of your citizenship responsibilities within a self-governing medical staff. But for those who do more, if you can define what that scope of work is, you can develop a fair compensation mechanism. This may be based on time spent or on tasks performed. You can pay for meeting attendance if the meeting is seen as burdensome because of preparation requirements. If someone is a paid medical director and the expectation is that part of his or her responsibilities is to review physician care, you may wish to exclude this person from receiving additional payment for carrying out quality improvement initiatives.

Who should pay? Typically, the hospital will be the source of compensation. Sometimes the hospital may provide the medical staff with a lump sum of funds to pay physicians for various activities and let the medical staff determine the precise distribution. Or the medical staff will provide some or all of the funds from medical staff dues. The latter two approaches work particularly well if the medical staff culture is suspicious of physicians who receive funds from the hospital. Whatever mechanism is used, it needs to be based on a consensus of the medical staff, the administration, and the board on the best approach.

How much should you pay? The legal issue here is based on the Stark Law for inurnment. You need to establish an administrative hourly rate for physicians and apply it equally to all physicians, regardless of specialty. Usually this rate is in the range of $75–$150 per hour. Then you need to establish a method to quantify the actual work being performed. You can either require the physician to track his or her actual time for reviewing cases or establish general per-case compensation. For example, if the average case review takes 30 minutes and your rate is $100 per hour, a physician reviewing three cases in a month would be paid $150.

This discussion should not be construed as an endorsement of paying physicians for peer review. If you choose to adopt this approach because it is right for your medical staff, this will help you evaluate the options.

PEER REVIEW: WHY DO WE NEED TO EVALUATE PHYSICIAN COMPETENCE?

Should Physicians Be Paid to Perform Peer Reviews?

Due to rising costs and tighter reimbursement, many physicians feel they need to spend as much time as they can on their individual practices. The challenge of balancing this time with a life outside of medicine means that many physicians are not willing to volunteer to participate in peer review activities, especially those that are inefficient and time-consuming.

Since the first edition of this book, this question has been raised by medical staff leaders and committee members more frequently than in the past. No physician will ever get rich from serving on a peer review committee. However, the increasing economic pressures on physicians to maintain high levels of productivity in their office practices and the desire for lifestyles that are less committed to the hospital has caused a decline in voluntary participation in peer review for many medical staffs.

The answer is not a simple one. It is based on a number of factors, including to what degree your medical staff culture will even accept payment of physicians for performing administrative tasks. As you look to create an effective peer review program, it is important that you at least consider this issue. The box below provides questions and approaches that can help you make a decision that best suits your medical staff.

Physician Leader–Driven Peer Review: A Medical Staff Leader's View

Note: The following is a speech by Dr. Michael McNamara given at High Point Regional Health System at the quarterly medical staff meeting in January 2006. Dr. McNamara was the incoming chair of the new medical staff peer review committee, redesigned as the central multi-specialty committee and titled the professional improvement committee. He was asked to acquaint the staff with the purpose of the reformulated committee. I found his presentation particularly articulate and compelling and asked if I might share his thoughts in this book. Here are his remarks:

"For those of you who read the quarterly update, you know that our mission is to bring exceptional healthcare to the people of the area that we serve. I have some good news for you. We have already assembled and credentialed an exceptional medical staff at our hospital. Reflect on the many medical and surgical specialties that we represent. Think of how many thousands of hours of advanced training in residencies, fellowships, and continuing medical education are part of the science of medicine that we bring to bear. Reflect on our collective experience of managing thousands of cases of acute and chronic care and the lives saved, the thousands of surgeries performed and suffering eased, and

the thousands of new lives brought into the world with our hands. We are filled with the skills of the science of medicine.

"*And by training, choice, and inherent compassion, we bring the art of medicine to the bedside of the ill and suffering. Our empathy, our patience, and our skill of listening speak to the art of our profession. I think that we do it well, and we honor the profession. We don't employ a trade. We administer with gifts.*

"*We do well in the art and the science of medicine. But in the day-to-day practice of our skill, the profession of medicine, we may measure less well. Each of us brings with us to our medical duty and service the baggage of pressures each day. Lack of sleep, constraints of time to see more patients and make quicker judgments, the nagging pinch of diminishing reimbursements, demands on our time for the business of medicine grab an ugly hold. And many days we cannot leave behind our personal worries, be they financial, family, or failing health. Thus, there are days when each of us may function within our practice of medicine at a level that falls below what we expect of ourselves and of each other.*

"*We as a medical staff have a duty to measure our own performance. Should we fail to faithfully carry this out, someone else will step in and assess and measure us. We have the responsibility to keep the scales and balances of professional assessment in house. I have been asked to chair the professional improvement committee. This is the committee tasked to carry the scales and balances—to measure the staff with a plan to continually improve our professionalism. This implementation may not be easy.*

"*For those of you who feel that this committee is instituted to be critical, judgmental, and punitive, then I want you to know that my first job as chairman is to prove to you that you are wrong. This committee does receive, and will continue to receive, written requests to evaluate aspects of patient care when someone (patient, family of patient, hospital staff, or your professional peers) has concerns that the practice of the profession of the science and art of medicine failed their expectations, or failed their understanding of a perceived standard. We will ask you to give us information to enable us to make an evaluation. If there is no merit to the report, we will let you know. If there are system errors in this hospital that interfere with efficient professional practice, we will work to fix them. If you are a physician who through lack of sufficient training, personal arrogance, or honest error falls below the standard we hold ourselves to, then we will give encouragement and assistance, and if need be, outside intervention and training to help you lift your professionalism to better the collective us.*

"As I told the committee on our first meeting, we will succeed by that which we do not know. Our impact will be measured by the patient who does not die, the postoperative infection that never occurs, the length-of-stay outlier that goes home on time, and by being spared the blot of rancid community publicity for an event that never occurs.

"We are an intelligent group of men and women with great gifts of knowledge, compassion, and service, and we are capable of change. We can change for the worse, or we can change for the better. I'm counting on the better. We will need your help."

The privilege society has granted us to have a self-governing medical staff will only remain if medical staff leaders take on the responsibility of mutual accountability for physician performance that Dr. McNamara has so clearly articulated.

REFERENCE

1. Witherell v. Weimer, 85 Ill. 2d 146 [1981].

From Punitive to Positive: Creating a Performance Improvement Culture for Peer Review

We often define an organization's culture as its shared values and beliefs. But a culture is really defined by how people behave, which reveals their true values and beliefs. Thus, culture is not static; rather, it is re-created every day through people's actions.

Culture is also not a regulatory compliance issue. The regulatory standards for peer review can be met with either a punitive or a positive approach. Medical staff culture is ultimately a choice, either a conscious or de facto one, and institutions have no one but themselves to blame if the culture is not what they'd like it to be.

Therefore, as we try to define a medical staff peer review culture and either reinforce it or, if necessary, change it, we must first look at what we value and how we act. For example, do we say we value data, yet whenever it is provided, the discussion immediately focuses on its inaccuracies? Do we say we value collegiality, but send accusatory letters when inquiring about a case under review? Do we say we value excellence, but have set no targets to recognize it? Linking your actions to your values is the key to defining your culture.

Why should you care about your peer review culture? Culture is the soil into which you sow the seeds to obtain the harvest of physician improvement. If you sow the seeds in fertile soil, you will have success. If you sow into rocky soil, your efforts will yield little result.

Because each medical staff has its own culture, if you don't address the realities of that culture, attempts to improve the effectiveness of your peer review program may be met with profound resistance and, potentially, outright failure. For example, many medical staff leaders take solutions from other medical staffs and try to implement them directly in their own setting only to see them fail. This is because culture was not taken into account either in the design or change management strategy.

CHAPTER 2

How Can Culture Change?

A primary goal of this book is to help medical staffs move from a punitive or indifferent peer review culture to one that supports physician improvement and the pursuit of excellence. The good news is that peer review culture can indeed change. But how do you get there? In my experience of working with medical staffs, there are four requirements for successful cultural change.

The first requirement is physician leadership with a vision of better values. Unless physician leaders can articulate to the staff what they would like the culture to become and why, most people are not interested in change for change sake. Typically, the development of these values begins with the leader's recognition that peer review is perceived, or actually is, punitive. Through outside education, the physician leadership realizes that there is a better way. Communicating this new vision to the staff is essential but not always easy. Sometimes the leader may return from an education program on peer review and feel like Moses coming down with the tablets only to find the people dancing around the golden calf.

The second requirement is a process that defines the specific behaviors that demonstrate those values. This requires examination by a group of physician leaders and support staff of your peer review structure, processes, and data to align them with your values. The majority of this book will be devoted to that process.

The third requirement is strong physician leadership to drive the change management strategy. Unlike software that you download to your computer, ideas driving change generally are not self-implementing. As the physician members question the new approaches, physician leaders must demonstrate resolve to help the medical staff stay the course.

The fourth requirement is sufficient time to allow for the use and acceptance of change. Changing behaviors doesn't happen overnight. Just like moving from a traditional cellphone to a smartphone takes repetition over time to be able to successfully use all its features, a medical staff needs to use the new peer review "apps" to learn how they really work and how they can actually change in their culture. Typically, it takes approximately one to two years to see a lasting impact. By setting realistic expectations about the time frame for change, physician leaders avoid the "are we there yet?" syndrome with which parents on trips with small children are quite familiar.

Note that all of these requirements require engaged physician leadership. While there is tremendous value in having a strong support staff for peer review, physician leaders need to fully engage in all phases of any peer review redesign effort for it to be effective.

Values of a Performance Improvement–Focused Peer Review Culture

In working with hundreds of physician leaders to create a performance improvement–focused peer review culture, there are six values that seem to resonate most strongly. These values provide a guidepost for the specific behaviors discussed in this book. They are:

- **Fairness:** The structure and processes of peer review do not favor one individual or group over another and improvement methods are appropriate for the type of improvement opportunity.

- **Transparency:** The peer review process is explained to the medical staff and physicians have access to their own data.

- **Data-driven:** Data, rather than opinion, is used to help understand and improve physician performance. As W. Edwards Deming said, "In God we trust, all others must bring data."

- **Self-improvement:** Individuals are informed early in the evaluation cycle of a potential improvement opportunity and given the chance for self-improvement.

- **Collegiality:** Interactions are designed to communicate the desire for understanding of all sides of the issue and to foster a dialogue that leads to an accurate conclusion that is accepted by all parties.

- **Pursuit of excellence:** Peer review is not just about eliminating poor care to achieve mediocrity; it also is responsible for driving the achievement of excellence in the priority areas defined by medical leadership and the board.

For cultural values to be more than slogans or signs on a wall, one must act in a way that will make these values real. There are five key actions that can help drive performance improvement–focused peer review:

- Minimize bias

- Collegial communication

CHAPTER 2

- Recognize excellence in physician performance

- Data acceptance

- Create mutual accountability

Minimize bias

One of the key challenges in any evaluation of human performance is how to eliminate or reduce bias. If the goal of a performance evaluation is to be fair, then we must seek out any actions, intended or unintended, that would bias the results.

To understand how bias can ruin a good thing, think of building your dream vacation home. In southwestern Michigan, there are several areas with 75-foot clay bluffs overlooking Lake Michigan and a nice strip of beach down below as a buffer between the lake and the bluff. Years ago, these areas seemed like a perfect place for a vacation house, but in the 1970s, the lake level rose, the beach disappeared, and the waves crashed steadily against the base of the bluff. Over a few years, the erosion resulted in several expensive homes falling off the cliff.

Think of bias as the waves, culture as the bluffs, and the peer review system as the vacation home. If you allow bias to persist, it will steadily erode your peer review culture. And when a catastrophic event occurs, such as when a corrective action is inappropriately taken, the root cause is generally traced back to a lack of recognition that the peer review process was being consistently undermined in several ways over a period of time. To understand the effect of bias, let's first discuss types and sources of bias and then consider some methods to address it.

What is bias? It is a tendency or preference toward a particular perspective or result. It may be either a conscious or unconscious prejudice that is introduced into a process. It may be due to individual preferences, or a systematic error introduced into sampling or testing that encourages one outcome over another. Intended or not, bias undermines the reliability or accuracy of the result.

Because it is an intrinsic part of any type of measurement or judgment designed and implemented by human beings, unfortunately, bias probably can never be completely eliminated from any process. However, it can be reduced in order to improve upon the result. It is critical to make every effort to reduce potential bias in peer review because practitioners will only buy in to a process that they perceive as fair and credible.

There are three major types of bias that affect the peer review process. They are:

- Human nature–related bias

- Systematic bias

- Statistical bias

How can understanding these three types of bias help improve peer review? As mentioned earlier, although we can't completely eliminate peer review bias, we can mitigate it to minimize its effect in two ways:

- Look for bias in your structures, procedures, and results

- Manage bias through your policies and systems

Before we see how these two strategies can be applied, let's remember our definition of peer review discussed in Chapter 1. Since peer review is more than case review, we will be looking for mechanisms to reduce bias in the evaluation of individual cases and in the use of aggregate data. Outlined below is a brief explanation of the three types of bias and some of the ways to reduce bias in peer review.

Human nature–related bias

Human nature contributes to bias by allowing us to use psychological "shortcuts" to reduce complexity and ambiguity in the world. We all wish life were simpler, and our brains try to accommodate us by finding shortcuts to decisions by relying on past patterns of thinking. This enables us to provide a rational response within the context of a simpler and less-threatening world. There are two main types of bias related to human nature: group and personal bias.

Group bias is when a group of individuals has a shared set of beliefs or experiences that result in a relatively predictable way of thinking or responding. This concept of "groupthink" results in the group tending to accept information that meets its common paradigm and reject, or at least not consider, information that is contrary to how it thinks.

It is the lack of diversity in the group that can create this bias. To avoid a group bias, it is best to structure the group to ensure that other views are included. There are two types of group bias that tend to affect peer review: professional bias (e.g., physicians think differently than nurses) and specialty bias (e.g.,

REASONS FOR PERSONAL BIAS

Personal bias arises when there is a difference between our perception or opinion of a result and the actual result. This can manifest in the following ways:

- Fear of retribution from a colleague, either personally, professionally, or economically

- Fear that an adverse peer review judgment will have a negative effect on a colleague's professional and personal life

- Anger toward a competitor or colleague for a perceived wrong that deserves retribution

- Desire to protect or shield a colleague, partner, employer, and/or employee from potential damage to his or her reputation or standing

- Desire to protect or shield a group of individuals (e.g., department, division, private enterprise) from potential damage to reputation or standing

- Certainty regarding analysis despite subsequent evidence to the contrary (anchoring bias)

- Selective elimination of information that does not confirm an initial analysis or impression (confirmation bias)

- A tendency to base judgments on information that is readily available, most recent, or that contains strong emotional content (availability bias)

- Inadvertently linking current circumstances to patterns or perceptions established in the past (representative bias)

- Maintaining an irrational commitment toward an issue, despite mounting evidence to the contrary (escalation of commitment bias)

- Inappropriately ascribing a pattern to random events (randomness error or bias)

- The tendency to inappropriately surmise a decision or action based on retrospective analysis (e.g., "I would have handled it differently") (hindsight bias)

- And most commonly, the tendency to overestimate our ability to judge and analyze a situation correctly, despite evidence to the contrary (overconfidence bias) surgeons think differently than internists). One of the main reasons that many medical staffs have found multi-specialty peer review committees to be successful is that they reduce the likelihood of groupthink by bringing all perspectives to the table. This will be discussed in detail in Chapter 4.

Personal bias is our view of the world that is created by the sum of our individual experiences: where we grew up, our parents' values, and how our friends act. Although we might make conscious efforts to overcome personal bias, we all retain some degree of it as part of our individuality.

The key to minimizing personal bias is to minimize the effect of the individual on the final decision. The following are four ways you can achieve this outcome:

1. Design your peer review structure so that a committee, rather than an individual, makes the final determination. This is the reason our legal system uses a jury—the group cancels out the personal biases of the individual members. Although a good peer review process will use an initial individual reviewer for efficiency, the group should make the final decision.

2. Protect reviewer anonymity. People are more open to putting aside their personal biases when they know they will not be subject to personal retribution, real or imagined.

3. Improve inter-rater reliability. A major problem for peer review is the potential variance among reviewers because medical staffs fail to proactively seek to "calibrate" evaluations of individual cases or aggregate data.

4. Create and follow a strong conflict-of-interest policy. When individuals with potential conflicts are involved, the committee must be aware of these situations and handle them appropriately.

Systematic bias

Whenever someone is the subject of a formal evaluation, someone else has designed a system for that evaluation. Systematic bias occurs when flaws are present in the evaluation system that can influence the individuals responsible for the decision in a way that can lead to incorrect results. These flaws may be intended but most often the result of the "law of unintended consequences." This is where someone thought a particular approach would be beneficial or neutral and did not realize the hidden bias that was being introduced.

CHAPTER 2

Systematic bias in peer review can be found in the procedures used to evaluate cases and come to decisions. Although it might seem that these are issues of personal bias, if we design a system so that most people would fail, then it is the system that is at fault.

A common source of systematic bias may be due to inconsistencies in the case review process. When we evaluate medical staff peer review programs, we often find this critical process is not clearly defined/documented, which leads to variations in procedures between committees or reviewers or a lack of the protection of practitioner rights. This can lead to a perception of unfairness. These issues will be further addressed in Chapter 6.

Statistical bias

Evaluations relying on data can be influenced by statistical bias when the findings are influenced by errors related to validity, reliability, or accuracy of the data. Chapter 5 discusses these concepts and how they might influence an evaluation.

Sampling errors can also be a form of statistical bias if the sample is not robust enough to draw conclusions. For example, if a 5% sample audit is performed for procedure complications where the expected rate is less than 1%, it is unlikely that one will be able to determine whether an individual physician has any issues.

If you think of peer review as only chart review of individual cases based on review criteria, you might not think statistical bias plays much of a role. However, statistical bias has a tremendous influence, even on case review, because if you are not using the right measures for the questions you are asking, you will bias your results.

The first part of asking the right question is measuring issues that are relevant to physician performance. If physicians are not primarily responsible for the variance in a measure (e.g., patient falls), then it is not a valid measure of physician performance.

A second part of asking the right question is choosing the right type of measure. The Greeley Company has used an approach that classifies indicators into three types: review, rule, and rate. Using the wrong type of measure can bias the results. For example, using case review to evaluate known common procedural complications instead of measuring the complication rate is biased against the high-volume physician who may have more complications only by virtue of fact that he does more procedures. Chapter 5 further discusses the use of these indicator types.

A third source of systematic peer review bias is the reliability and accuracy of physician performance measures. This is driven mainly by physician attribution. If we don't identify the correct physician, we may come to the wrong conclusion. Although attribution is not a major problem for chart review, it can be a big problem for rate measures. Chapter 8 further discusses these issues.

Collegial communication

How we communicate with each other is an important expression of our cultural values. For example, if we use an aggressive tone in a letter requesting information about a case under review, it may create a defensive response. Taking the time to make sure our communication is collegial can make all the difference in the perception as to whether peer review is viewed as punitive or helpful. This applies to both written and verbal communication.

One helpful practice is to not start the peer review process by thinking in negative terms (e.g., "Why are you bad?"). Instead, begin with a more neutral view (e.g., "Why are you different?"). This allows your mind to be open to the possibility that there is a good explanation for the physician's decisions and actions. This approach applies to whether you are reviewing an individual case or looking at rate data that is exceeding a target.

A second helpful practice is to frame inquiries as two-part questions. Rather than asking, "Why did you not order insulin on admission?" one would ask, "Did you consider ordering insulin on admission and, if so, why did you choose not to?"

A third helpful practice is to create template letters that always explain the nature of the communication and recognize the limitations of the data. For example, in a letter of inquiry, after asking the physician questions about your concerns, the following paragraph is often helpful:

"We recognize the medical record often does not contain all the information needed to evaluate care in a complex case. Prior to the committee making a determination on the case, we would like to have your input in writing to the above questions to more fully understand the care provided to this patient."

Often, communication about physician performance is sent by the quality staff and may have a rather business-like tone. This is not done with ill intent, but rather the quality staff does not recognize the cultural impact of the communication on physicians. Since it is the medical staff's culture that will be affected, physician leaders must be actively involved in designing the standard-type letters used in peer review.

Recognize excellence in physician performance

For peer review to be balanced, it must recognize all levels of physician performance, not just poor performance. Part of a performance improvement culture is the desire to pursue excellence, not just to be comfortable with average or mediocre performance. Many physicians have this goal as a personal desire but believe that it is not their responsibility to make this a goal of the medical staff. Other physicians have expressed the belief that we are expected to do excellent work so there is no need for additional recognition. By these choices, they may not realize that they are perpetuating a negative element in their peer review culture.

Despite the belief that physicians don't need praise (perhaps a vestige of the older generation of physicians), a Greeley Company culture survey of medical staffs finds that appreciation is rated as the lowest cultural attribute. It is long past time to move to a model that treats physicians as typical human beings that respond well to deserved recognition.

Recognition of excellence can be done in the case review process by identifying and sending letters to physicians commending them for exemplary practices. It can also be done in the use of aggregate data for ongoing professional practice evaluation (OPPE) by setting targets for excellent performance in addition to targets for follow-up. These approaches will be discussed further in Chapters 6 and 9.

Data acceptance

Currently, healthcare is awash in a sea of data. However, for many medical staffs, getting physicians to accept and use performance data has been a struggle. Many hospitals have physician-level data but have not distributed it to their physicians or used it for OPPE out of fear of attack on the accuracy of the data. Others have not invested in obtaining it because they are concerned it will not be used. Unfortunately, this anti-data attitude ultimately is detrimental to physicians because without data they are unaware of improvement opportunities or achievement of excellence.

Although the availability and use of physician data seems like a technical issue based on information systems and data accuracy and reliability, fundamentally it is a cultural issue. Unless a medical staff creates a culture of data acceptance, all the information technology advances will go for naught. For example, I have seen that a number of hospitals that purchased physician data systems that allow all physicians direct data access found that unless they had a strong data acceptance culture, only a few physicians actually looked at their data.

FROM PUNITIVE TO POSITIVE: CREATING A PERFORMANCE IMPROVEMENT CULTURE FOR PEER REVIEW

Ironically, physicians as a group are scientists and tend to like data. So what is the problem? While physicians may raise strong concerns about data accuracy (many of which have validity), their real concern is data use. That is where the cultural issue comes into play. Remember, culture is defined by behaviors. So which behaviors define your culture?

In punitive culture, the typical response to data is to challenge it and fight to the death to be sure it is not used. In a performance improvement culture, the physician response to data is to seek to understand it, even with its flaws, to be sure that any improvement opportunity is not missed.

Leaders in a punitive peer review culture see data as the end point and have a tendency to move directly from data to action. Leaders in an improvement-focused culture see data as a starting point for discussion with the physician to find out why he or she is different. It provides the basis for further understanding of the data and assisting the physician to improve.

How do you create this culture? Here are some specific behaviors that will reinforce a data-acceptance culture:

- Create medical staff policies that clearly define how data will be evaluated before conclusions are reached that may affect a physician's practice and reputation. (This will be discussed in Chapter 8.)

- Give physicians their data, warts and all, so they can get used to it, understand it, and begin to self-correct. Ironically, not giving physicians their data out of fear of a negative reaction perpetuates the physicians' fear of the data.

- Acknowledge data imprecision. This approach reduces some of a physician's natural defensiveness. When data comes out of a computer and has multiple decimal places, there is often a tendency to believe the data is more precise than it really is. We call this the "illusion of precision." Also, physician attribution accuracy is highly dependent on data collection systems that were often designed to capture financial rather than clinical data.

- Engage the medical staff in selecting competency measures. It is critical that physicians understand and are involved in the details of the measurement process. The saying "The devil is in the details" is never truer than when it comes to defining useful performance measures. As we will discuss in Chapter 4, there are a number of issues to consider when selecting useful measures of physician performance.

- Educate the medical staff on physician competency reports. Although education alone doesn't change culture, it is a necessary component of effective change-management strategies. Medical staff leaders involved in the development of the physician competency reports should understand their goals and uses and then educate the medical staff. If not, the majority of the medical staff will find them unfamiliar and may resist or resent the use of such reports.

Create mutual accountability: The physician performance pyramid

Organizations do not achieve outstanding results by accident—they take a powerful, commonsense approach that motivates all employees to do their best consistently. The Walt Disney Company uses this approach to get every single staff member in its theme parks to be uniformly nice, upbeat, and helpful, from the people behind the concession counters to the ticket takers, to those dressed up like Disney® characters. Luxury hotels such as The Ritz-Carlton® apply this approach to provide outstanding service every day.

Each of these exceptional organizations applies an approach that promotes outstanding individual performance. This approach is called the performance pyramid (see Figure 2.1). At its core it is a human resources management tool. It has been taught for years by the American College of Physician Executives, and The Greeley Company has successfully pioneered applying this model to hospital medical staffs. Since peer review essentially is the human resource department of the medical staff, it should not be surprising that applying human resource approaches can improve the effectiveness of peer review.

The pyramid is composed of layers. Each layer represents an essential responsibility that physician leaders should carry out in order to optimize physician performance. The model is designed in the shape of a pyramid because the more time leaders spend on the base layers, the less time they will need to spend on the upper layers with the distasteful tasks of managing poor performance and taking corrective action. Let's discuss the six layers of the pyramid and the role of each in improving physician performance.

Appoint excellent physicians

If you start by bringing people into the hospital who are well qualified and appropriate for your medical staff, you improve your ability to achieve the level of excellence you desire. For example, consider Walt Disney Company employees. Why are they so polite and friendly? It's not simply because Disney

FROM PUNITIVE TO POSITIVE: CREATING A PERFORMANCE IMPROVEMENT CULTURE FOR PEER REVIEW

2.1 Power of the Pyramid—Achieving Great Physician Performance

- Take corrective action
- Manage poor performance
- Provide periodic feedback
- Measure actual performance
- Set and communicate expectations
- Appoint excellent physicians

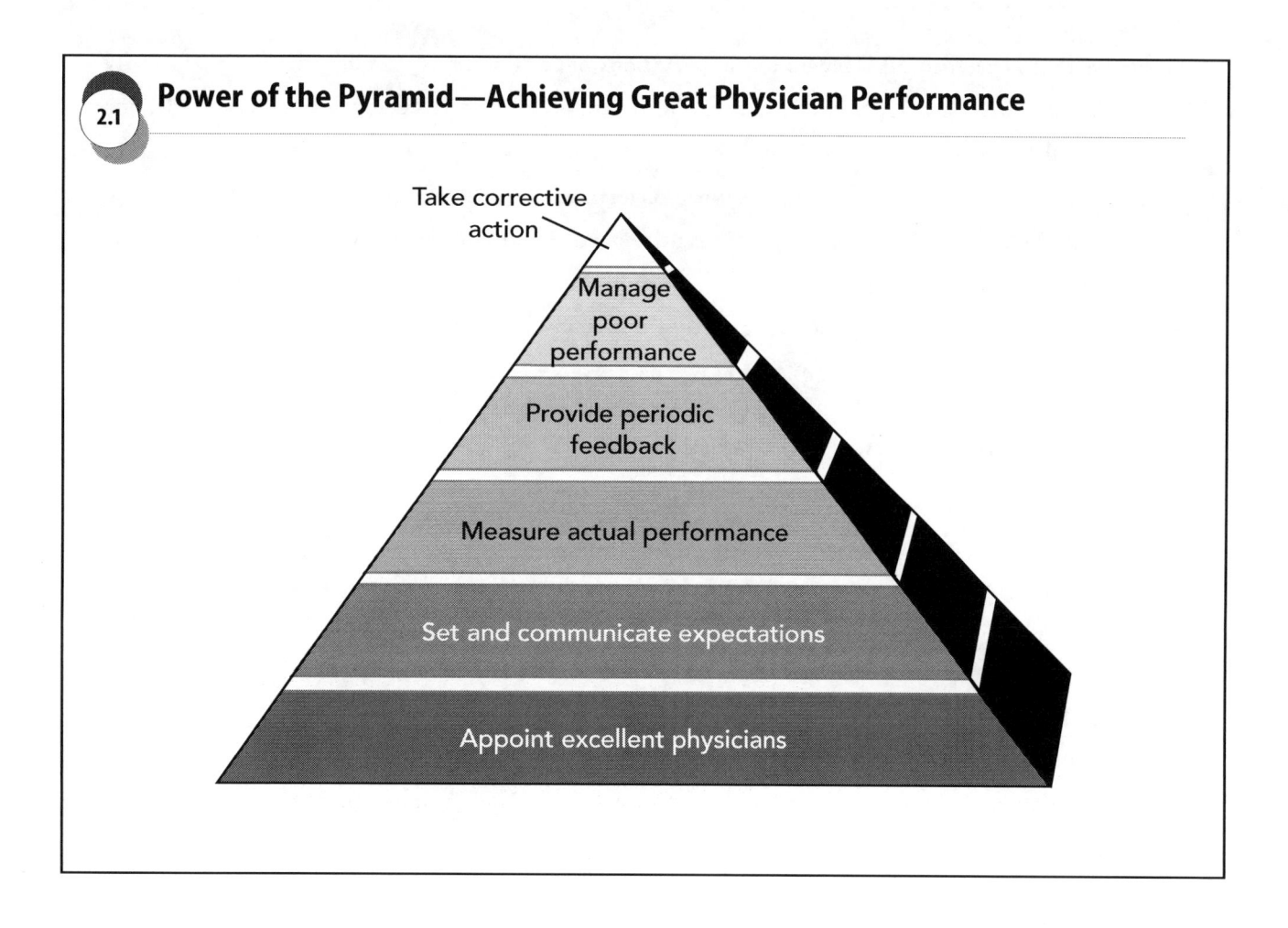

trains them to be so but rather because the company carefully selects people who have these attributes in the first place. Thus, careful selection is the essence of the first layer.

To select physicians carefully, you must adopt solid credentialing and privileging systems. This means going beyond the minimum required federal, state, and regulatory requirements to create and maintain the highest possible standards for medical staff appointment. Require applicants to demonstrate excellent previous clinical performance, to provide superior professional references, and to demonstrate the ability to relate well to colleagues and other employees.

Set and communicate expectations

Medical staff often do not set and communicate expectations for physicians very well. For example, a new physician who has just admitted a patient might want to obtain a consult with another staff member. How should the physician do so? Is it acceptable to write an order on a chart and expect the

The key is that physicians must have these expectations of each other as members of a democratically organized, self-governing body that reports to the hospital board of trustees. Medical staff leadership should tell all new physicians, in writing, what is expected of them if they are to achieve excellence at that hospital. This one- to two-page document is a statement of the culture of the medical staff, or "how we do things here," and serves as an executive summary of all the bylaws, rules and regulations, and policies and procedures. These expectations are best organized around a physician performance framework. The six core competencies are the most common current framework. In Chapter 7, we will outline the six steps you must take to set these expectations.

Measure performance against expectations

Once a hospital has established expectations and communicated them to the medical staff, it must measure each physician's performance against those expectations.

The basic premise that measurement drives improvement is the foundation of any successful quality program—that is, if you can't measure it, you can't manage it. Therefore, once physician performance indicators are established, medical staff leaders must ensure that all physicians know that their performance will be measured, how it will be measured, and how it will be compared to that of their peers. Chapter 5 discusses how to develop physician performance indicators in detail. Again, the six core competencies will help drive the use of expectation-based measurement and will assist medical staffs to move away from the more random approach of picking performance measures based merely on data availability.

Provide periodic feedback

Physicians do not really know whether they are meeting expectations unless they receive periodic feedback regarding their performance. And when they receive it in a timely and easy-to-follow manner, they can use this feedback for self-improvement.

Providing feedback with the opportunity for self-improvement is the cornerstone of a peer-review performance improvement culture. Chapter 11 addresses performance feedback in more detail. The OPPE requirements for systematic evaluation of physician performance data can best be met by creating routine feedback so that the individual physician and the medical staff leaders can evaluate the data together.

FROM PUNITIVE TO POSITIVE: CREATING A PERFORMANCE IMPROVEMENT CULTURE FOR PEER REVIEW

PEER REVIEW MONTHLY: "AMAZING GRACE"

Today, my wife and I celebrate our 32nd wedding anniversary. The primary reason that our marriage has lasted this long, especially in light of my many flaws, can be attributed to my wife's ability to demonstrate grace (she has many other wonderful attributes, but due to limitations of space, I will focus on just this one).

The best definition I have heard for grace is "unmerited favor." It means having the ability to accept and, yes, even forgive, people despite their flaws. While a marriage starts with love, I believe it is sustained by grace.

What does this have to do with peer review, the topic of this monthly column? Well, it got me thinking about the similarities between a successful marriage and a successful medical staff peer review program. Despite all the technicalities of regulations and procedures, like marriage, peer review is a relationship marked by mutual accountability that can be approached punitively or with grace.

The key here is to start with the understanding that, as members of the medical staff, you are mutually accountable for the evaluation and improvement of the quality and safety of the care that you provide individually in the hospital setting. That's what you agree to when you sign the bylaws and say "I do."

Then, like in a marriage, we begin to realize and understand the expectations we have for each other. Some of these are clear upfront (e.g., "Don't leave the seat up" or "Complete your medical records"). Some expectations evolve over time based on the changing world around us and our own changing needs and perspectives. Medical staffs have historically given physician competency a technical definition, but now we recognize that multiple competencies define an excellent physician, including skills in the areas of communication and systems-based practice.

Ultimately, our medical staff relationship, like a marriage, is defined by our behaviors and our response to feedback, especially in light of changing expectations. In medical staff terms we call this peer review. (I am not sure if there is a marriage term but anyone who has been married knows the process does happen.) This is where grace comes in. How we give that feedback and help an individual understand and deal with their shortcomings can be done punitively or with some measure of grace, particularly if the individual is willing to listen and change.

Does this mean peer review should never lead to corrective action? Just as some marriages can't work if one or both parties are unwilling to even try to meet the other's expectations and needs, there are some medical staff members who are unwilling to recognize the need for improvement and must be dealt with in stricter terms that may result in ending the relationship. But before we get there, let's be sure we extended as much grace as possible to keep the relationship whole.

Editor's Note: This article was originally published in Medical Staff Leader Insider, July 1, 2009.

Manage poor performance

If feedback does not result in self-improvement, appropriate leaders or mentors should meet with the physician to discuss improvement strategies. These leaders or mentors should help motivate the physician to change or eliminate unacceptable performance and should monitor the physician's progress. Medical staff leaders should not wait until reappointment to address performance issues—rather, they should discuss such issues with the appropriate physician as soon as concerns arise. However, please note that managing poor performance is not the same as corrective action.

This layer of the pyramid is the most uncomfortable for physician leaders who have not been trained to carry it out collegially and effectively. Therefore, physician leaders often avoid such confrontations until seriously negative data forces them to act, but such avoidance is unfair to the physician and dangerous to patients. Because this is such an important issue, physician performance management for peer review will be discussed in more depth in Chapter 10.

Take corrective action

Medical staff leadership must act when all of the aforementioned steps have been taken but a physician fails to self-improve and his or her poor performance threatens the quality of patient care.

Such action is known as corrective action and is a formal process that involves loss of membership or privileges. Legal counsel should become involved at the first sign that a formal corrective action is necessary or is likely to be necessary. In extreme situations, complete termination of medical staff membership and privileges might be necessary, but sometimes it is possible to change or limit the scope of a physician's practice to correct the situation.

Peer Review and the Just Culture

A discussion about creating a positive culture for peer review would be incomplete without recognizing the concept of the Just Culture created by David Marx[1]. This concept was developed for creating a positive patient safety culture, in particular, to fairly define culpability for potential or actual harm involving medication errors. A number of organizations are either looking at this concept to determine its applicability to peer review or have begun to apply it.

Although it is beyond the scope of this book to fully develop a Just Culture–based approach to peer review, a few preliminary thoughts may be useful relative to how this concept fits with the concepts and strategies introduced in this book. Overall, the Just Culture ideas are very synergistic with the performance improvement focus of this book. For example, the pyramid seeks to provide feedback to educate and allow for self-improvement performance; the Just Culture also encourages self-reporting for unintended errors to enhance learning, and encourages counseling for negligence that is not part of a recurring problem. Also, the use of rule indicators described in Chapter 5 is synergistic with the Just Culture because it treats minimal events through educational feedback with no consequences unless a pattern emerges.

The Just Culture is based on a combination of legal concepts of negligence with corporate approaches regarding culpability or fault related to safety in high-risk industries, such as aviation, that have an impact on employee morale and function. The goal of the Just Culture is to assign the consequences for an unsafe act in a fair way based on an understanding of an individual's accountability and responsibilities within the context of the systems and circumstances that the individual was operating.

The Just Culture is not a blame-free culture. It merely tries to provide a consistent guide to determine 1) when a person is truly at fault for a specific act and 2) what the reasonable consequences are for that individual that will best serve the individual's and the organization's interests in the long run.

The four key categories of the Just Culture for assigning fault are as follows:

1. Human Error: Unintended slips, lapses, and mistakes

2. Negligent Conduct: Failure to exercise care expected of a prudent worker

3. Reckless Conduct: Conscious disregard for a known risk

4. Knowing Violations: Conscious disregard for known rules

To guide managers and organizations in making fair decisions, algorithms have been developed using these concepts. These algorithms typically ask a series of questions:

1. Were the actions intended?

2. Was the person under the influence of unauthorized substances?

3. Did the person knowingly violate existing policies, procedures, or expectations?

4. Would another person in the same situation perform in the same manner?

5. Does this person have a history of unsafe acts?

Based on the answers to those questions, the actions taken may involve consoling, coaching, counseling, progressive discipline, termination, or system changes.

The Just Culture was developed on an employee-based model for medication errors. Given this background, how have the Just Culture concepts been applied to peer review?

Since it is primarily event-based, the Just Culture approach has been most often applied to case review. In our discussion with organizations applying it, they have used it after the committee has rated the physician's care as less than appropriate. They then apply the Just Culture algorithm to determine the best approach for improvement or corrective action.

REFERENCE

1. Marx, David. *Patient Safety and the 'Just Culture': A Primer for Health Care Executives,* The Trustees of Columbia University; New York, 2001.

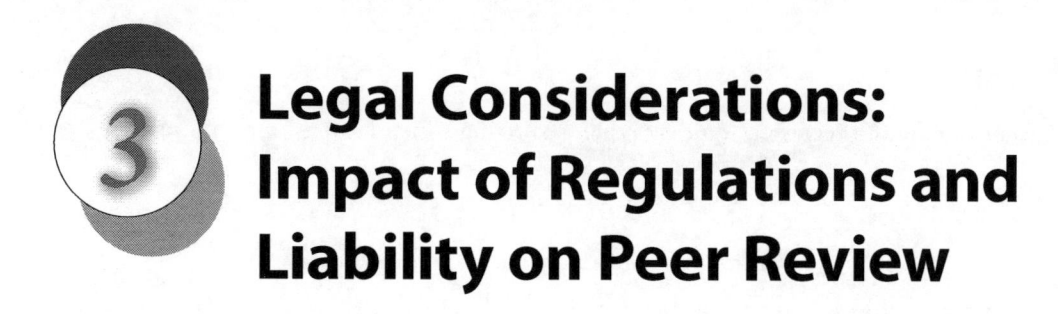

3. Legal Considerations: Impact of Regulations and Liability on Peer Review

In earlier editions of this book, the focus of this chapter was entirely on The Joint Commission. Since The Joint Commission is still the major accreditor, it is still a major focus of this book. However, with more options for accreditation today and with closer ties between the Centers for Medicare & Medicaid Services (CMS) standards and The Joint Commission, it is important to address how the accreditation organization model specifically affects the accreditation requirements for peer review.

While the Joint Commission standards reflect the CMS *Conditions of Participation (CoP)*, the standards, language, numbering, and survey process do not directly follow the *CoP*. Other accrediting bodies with deemed status, such as Healthcare Facilities Accreditation Program (HFAP), Det Norske Veritas (DNV), or state departments of health more faithfully follow the *CoP* framework.

So how do the requirements for peer review differ? We will first discuss The Joint Commission's approach and then compare that to the *CoP* accreditation models.

Redefining Peer Review: OPPE, FPPE, and the Core Competencies

In its 2007 medical staff standards, The Joint Commission placed a renewed emphasis on the relationship between peer review and the credentialing and privileging processes. Although it adopted some new terms designed to clarify what peer review should accomplish, many concepts that these standards promote have always been there. In the past, however, these standards were not strongly enforced.

There were basically two changes to the 2007 Joint Commission medical staff standards that affect physician performance measurement. The first change was the adoption of a comprehensive framework defining the dimensions of physician performance for which medical staff physicians with clinical privileges should be held accountable. These are called the general or core competency expectations for physicians (mentioned in Chapter 1). In adopting this framework, The Joint Commission has defined physician competency as more than a technical quality issue, requiring measurement in all these areas of competence.

However, there have been some challenges for medical staffs trying to comply with this new framework. For example, the general competencies framework itself was designed for physicians in a training setting, rather than those in active practice. As a result, the field has struggled to determine how to measure practice-based learning and subsequently The Joint Commission dropped the requirement for OPPE data for this category.

To help you begin to understand and apply these general competencies, Chapter 7 provides an in-depth look at each competency, and discusses the implications for physician performance measurement.

The second change is in how The Joint Commission has classified the approach to measurement of the competencies in that framework. These approaches are now labeled as ongoing professional practice evaluation (OPPE) and focused professional practice evaluation (FPPE). Although the general competencies will drive what is actually measured, the OPPE and FPPE standards focus on how data is used to evaluate and take action regarding physician performance. First, let's clarify the terms.

Ongoing professional practice evaluation

When the term OPPE is mentioned, most medical staffs automatically think in terms of a physician data profile. While the OPPE profile is an important output of it, OPPE is much broader than that. OPPE is the process for the routine measurement and evaluation of current competency for current medical staff members. Thus, it encompasses the main functions of a medical staff peer review program to establish routine measures or indicators of physician performance. While case review is still part of OPPE, an organization cannot successful meet the OPPE standards with case review alone.

OPPE has two main goals. The first is to obtain aggregate data for the general competencies that can make peer review evaluation more systematic and objective. The second is to make physician performance evaluation more timely so that trends are identified as an ongoing activity, not just at reappointment every two years. The second goal also provides opportunities to improve the individual performance prior to the reappointment decision.

Therefore, although OPPE may appear to be regulatory-driven, it is perfectly suited for a performance improvement-focused peer review program. In fact, as a best-practice approach, The Greeley Company had been helping medical staffs to implement semi-annual monitoring of feedback of physician performance data for over five years before the OPPE standards were developed.

LEGAL CONSIDERATIONS: IMPACT OF REGULATIONS AND LIABILITY ON PEER REVIEW

The primary goal of this book is to help medical staffs develop a practical approach to OPPE that adheres to a comprehensive framework and has a measurable impact on improving physician performance on an ongoing basis.

Focused professional practice evaluation

The term FPPE has caused some confusion because it applies to two types of evaluations. I have compared this confusion to how former heavyweight boxing champion George Foreman named all five of his sons George. He also gave each son a unique nickname. So why not just give each boy a different name from the start? Although The Joint Commission has not modified the terms, a number of organizations have created some nicknames (e.g., "Monk," "Big Wheel," "Red," and "Little Joey") to keep them straight. The key is when someone says FPPE, always ask, "Which FPPE do you mean?"

The first form of FPPE, so-called initial FPPE, is the evaluation of new medical staff members or current members with new privileges for a focused period of time. This is done routinely and may be referred to as proctoring. The "focus" is for a defined period of time or number of patients needed to obtain this data. The goal is to obtain data to ensure that the physician is indeed competent to perform those privileges in your own setting. Unlike the second form of FPPE, this is not driven by any concern regarding physician competency.

This form of FPPE is performed in the first few months of the initiation of the privileges and is linked closely to the initial credentialing function. As such, it will not be addressed in detail in this book. While some of the data from OPPE may be used for initial FPPE, it is looked at sooner than the typical OPPE six-month cycle.

The second form of FPPE is linked to OPPE. Here the focus of the evaluation occurs because of either a concern raised by OPPE data or a need for focused monitoring as part of the improvement process. This is not anything really new: medical staff leaders have always followed up on concerns. This process of follow-up was in the standards prior to the term FPPE being applied to it.

So how does this all fit together? The OPPE-FPPE equation looks like this:

Effective Peer Review = Systematic Measurement (OPPE) + Systematic Evaluation (OPPE and FPPE) + Systematic Follow-through (FPPE).

This book will explore practical ways to make this equation work for your medical staff.

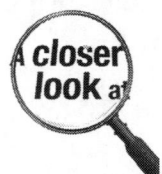

A closer look at: Focused Review of a Physician's Performance (FPPE)

A focused review is an intensive peer review of a physician's performance triggered by a concern related to any of the general competencies. Such reviews may be as innocuous as a retrospective chart review of specific procedures or as intensive as having a proctor observe a physician's patient care.

The Joint Commission requires medical staffs to define the circumstances that trigger a focused review. For example, when hospital performance improvement indicators show that a particular physician has aberrant data, the medical staff must conduct such a review. Medical staff leaders also must conduct a review when informed of poor physician performance—when, for instance, the physician has a "bad" case or a string of adverse patient outcomes, or when nurses notify medical staff leaders of their concerns regarding a physician's patient care activities.

The focused review process triggered by such circumstances must be flexible. Some quality issues are best investigated through retrospective chart reviews; others require that the organization appoint a proctor to observe the physician. Likewise, in some cases, the department chair can perform the review, but in others a medical staff member, outside expert, or physician panel must do so.

The Joint Commission requires a hospital to define when an external peer review is necessary. For example, consider using an outside expert when the department chair cannot or may not objectively evaluate the performance of a medical staff member. Such an expert also could intervene when the requested privileges are state-of-the-art and the medical staff members are unable to evaluate the credentials necessary to perform such procedures.

The focused review policy must state the time frame for the review. In addition, the physician under review should be permitted to participate in the process although the standards do not mandate any specific level of participation. Therefore, depending on the circumstances, the process may permit the physician to participate actively in the focused review or it may limit the physician to providing comments on the final report.

The Joint Commission also requires hospitals to have a method by which they select review panels for specific circumstances.

How the Standards Apply

Several Joint Commission medical staff (MS) standards are associated with aspects of peer review. Additionally, the performance improvement standards indirectly address peer review by discussing the management of sentinel events. However, not all sentinel events are associated with physician performance, and not all medical errors by physicians result in sentinel events.

LEGAL CONSIDERATIONS: IMPACT OF REGULATIONS AND LIABILITY ON PEER REVIEW

MS.06.01.05–MS.06.01.07: Granting, renewal, and revision of privileges

These standards require a hospital to have ongoing processes in place for granting, renewing, or revising criteria-based privileges. Among other things, this means you must develop criteria to determine whether an applicant can provide, or can continue to provide, patient care treatment and services within the scope of the privileges requested. The Joint Commission specifically states that these criteria should include evidence of current competence and peer recommendations when required.

It also requires that OPPE information be factored into the decision to maintain, revise, or revoke existing privileges prior to or at the time of renewal (MS.08.01.02). This now applies not only to physicians but to advanced practice professionals (APP) as well. The application of this to APPs is becoming a source of difficulty for medical staffs since often information systems do not attribute care to APPs.

The elements of performance for this point out that each reappraisal also should include information regarding a physician's professional performance, including clinical and technical skills and information from hospital performance improvement activities, when such data is available. Much of this information will come from the ongoing peer review processes outlined in this book.

MS.06.01.03: General competencies

The general competencies are a recommended framework for evaluating physician performance. If your medical staff uses a different framework, and you can explain how it covers the same areas as the six general competencies, it typically is accepted by The Joint Commission. However, because of the more universal acceptance of the general competencies over the past few years, we are seeing fewer medical staffs use a different framework.

MS.08.01.01: Focused reviews of a practitioner's performance

In addition to describing the general processes for reviewing a physician's performance, The Joint Commission has a specific standard that addresses focused reviews, specifically reviews by peers that physicians have traditionally called peer reviews. The Joint Commission makes it clear that this review is to be conducted by peers. However, the goal of The Joint Commission's focused review is not disciplinary. As is the goal of this book, The Joint Commission's goal is to improve physician performance. Information gathered as a result of focused reviews is to be integrated into performance improvement initiatives within the hospital.

Sentinel events and performance improvement

In the *Comprehensive Accreditation Manual for Hospitals,* The Joint Commission defines a sentinel event as "an unexpected occurrence involving death or serious physical or psychological injury, or the risk thereof." The performance improvement standards require hospitals to collect data so that they can monitor performance and systematically aggregate and analyze data, including identifying undesirable patterns or trends in performance. Hospitals also must have specific processes in place to identify and manage sentinel events, including processes to conduct root cause analysis (RCA) of sentinel events.

As noted earlier, peer review is not the same as RCA, although a sentinel event could trigger an individual case peer review. Similarly, some of the data gathered, aggregated, and analyzed in the context of overall performance improvement can be useful in measuring physician performance.

The CoP accreditation models

As mentioned at the start of this chapter, other accrediting body standards more closely align with the CMS *CoP*. While a detailed review of those standards is beyond the scope of this book, there is one key issue regarding how they address peer review.

First, while the *CoP* require a peer review process to evaluate physician competency, it does not define as explicitly as The Joint Commission how it must be done. For example, there are no standards describing a competency framework, ongoing evaluation, time frames for data review, or the types of data needed. The good news is this gives the organization a great deal of flexibility. The bad news is that it can make the accreditation survey more surveyor-dependent.

What the *CoP* do require is that you have policies and procedures that define how you can determine that a physician is competent and that you follow these policies. That means that your policies must make sense. For example, if you decided that your policy was that only subjective evaluations would be used to determine physician competency and physician performance data was not needed, the surveyor would have the right to raise the question as to whether that would really give you adequate information to make that decision. If you had data and only looked at it every two years, the surveyor could raise the question as to whether that would be frequent enough to be aware of trends.

The bottom line for those organizations that are not Joint Commission–accredited is that the OPPE/FPPE approach to peer review is well recognized and easily defensible in the face of a *CoP*-type survey. It is also well aligned with a performance improvement–focused peer review culture. Therefore, many organizations adopt this approach, along with other practices in this book, regardless of their accreditor.

Peer Review Protection Laws

There are three types of peer review protection laws: those granting immunity from lawsuits to persons and institutions, those declaring peer review work products to be privileged and inadmissible in court, and those allowing information related to peer reviews to remain confidential. These laws affect lawsuits brought by physician-plaintiffs and patient-plaintiffs.

For example, if a physician plaintiff's lawsuit involves, among other things, some aspect of the peer review process, the physician usually names everyone involved in the process in an attempt to find a "deep pocket." The physician-plaintiff will typically allege due-process violations, violations of the antitrust laws, defamation, or tortuous interference with a business relationship, and he or she will seek monetary damages. Likewise, a patient who is suing may name the same deep-pocket defendants and allege negligent credentialing. Even if the physician is the only person named as a defendant, the patient-plaintiff still may seek information from the peer review process to support the malpractice claim.

Remember that peer review statutes do not actually prevent a plaintiff from filing a lawsuit. Basically, anybody who has enough money to pay filing fees can file a lawsuit. Although the suit may be dismissed immediately, it still will have been filed, which can be very distressing for anyone named in it.

Physician peer reviewers also should note that a hospital's insurance policy typically covers all good-faith peer review participants and, thus, would cover any suits filed—even frivolous ones. "Covering them" includes providing a legal defense for individually named physician peer reviewers and coverage in the event that monetary damages are assessed, which is almost never. Hospital professional liability policies do not—nor should they—cover purposeful discriminatory or antitrust behavior.

Immunity addresses physicians' and hospitals' fears that they could be found liable for significant monetary damages in defamation, antitrust, or negligent credentialing lawsuits. The federal government and all state governments have passed immunity statutes of some kind.

CHAPTER 3

The Health Care Quality Improvement Act of 1986

The Health Care Quality Improvement Act of 1986 (HCQIA) grants immunity to healthcare professionals who engaged in good-faith evaluation of their peers. To qualify for federal immunity, however, the peer review decision must be a professional review action taken by a professional review body (see definitions in the box below). Moreover, the professional review action must have been taken:

- Based on the reasonable belief that the action was in furtherance of quality healthcare

- After a reasonable effort to obtain the facts of the matter

- After adequate notice and hearing procedures were afforded to the physician involved or after such other procedures as were fair to the physician under the circumstances

- Based on the reasonable belief that the action was warranted by the facts known, after such reasonable effort to obtain facts, and after meeting the statute's specific requirements for hearings

The HCQIA further states that professional review actions will be legally presumed to have met these four "safe harbor" provisions unless proven otherwise by a "preponderance of the evidence."

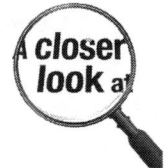

A closer look at

HCQIA definitions

The HCQIA defines a professional review action as "an action or recommendation of a professional review body which is taken or made in the conduct of professional review activity, which is based on the competence or professional conduct of an individual physician (which conduct affects or could affect adversely the health or welfare of a patient or patients), and which affects (or may affect) adversely the clinical privileges, or membership in a professional society, of the physician."

The HCQIA defines a professional review body as a "committee of a health care entity which conducts professional review activity, and includes any committee of the medical staff of such an entity when assisting the governing body in a professional review activity."

LEGAL CONSIDERATIONS: IMPACT OF REGULATIONS AND LIABILITY ON PEER REVIEW

State immunity laws

The majority of state statutes provide peer reviewers immunity from civil liability. The strongest statutes give immunity to all peer review committee members and to institutions and persons furnishing information to the committee; weaker statutes give immunity for only a few or for specified people. Note that the immunity is not absolute. As with the HCQIA, most states have qualified their grant of immunity. Many require the peer review action to have been taken without malice or in good faith.

Protection from discovery

The second type of protection is the work-product privilege, which prevents information associated with the peer review process from being discovered. This protection is based on the idea that physicians won't candidly discuss a colleague's shortcomings if their statements later could be discovered in judicial proceedings. All of the states, as well as the District of Columbia, recognize some form of privilege that protects various records and documents created as part of the peer review process. The HCQIA does not protect peer review documents from federal discovery.

State laws differ on which documents they protect. For example, some states protect "the reports, statements, memoranda, proceedings, findings, and other records of peer review committees or officers" but don't protect records given to the committee. Another state law allows discovery of materials produced out of sight of the peer review process. At the other end of the continuum are states that protect all information considered by the entity acting in a quality assurance process and that treat the records of such consideration as confidential.

In many states, the courts or the legislature have carved out areas in which the confidentiality provisions do not apply. It is not uncommon, for example, to find exceptions to the confidentiality provisions when a physician challenges his or her own peer review process.

Patient safety organizations and peer review protection

In 2005, the federal government passed legislation to allow protection of information from discovery of documents and data related to quality improvement entitled the Patient Safety and Quality Improvement Act, which went into effect in 2009. This legislation allowed healthcare organizations to form or participate in patient safety organizations (PSO). The PSO goal is to promote the aggregation and sharing of quality information to improve patient care without fear of its use in legal proceedings. While it is beyond the scope of this book to fully explore the details of the PSO, the potential impact on peer review is worthy of discussion.

The key protection participating in a PSO offers for peer review is that one can designate documents other than patient records (e.g., case review findings, letters of inquiry) as patient safety work products (PSWP). PSWP documents receive federal protection from discoverability rather than the state protection discussed earlier. Thus, the PSWP approach is particularly helpful in states where peer review protection has been weakened either by statute (e.g., Florida Amendment 7) or case law (e.g., Kentucky).

So why wouldn't everyone want to use the PSO approach to obtain federal protection for peer review? The problem with the PSWP designation is that in return for protection from discoverability, a PSWP cannot be used in an action against an individual. Thus, if a case review finding of inappropriate care were designated as a PSWP, it could not be used in a corrective action or fair hearing. The medical staff would have to redo the review process and not designate the documents as PSWPs. For this reason, despite the initial fervor to apply the PSO concept to peer review, hospitals in only the few states with significant problems with discoverability have chosen that approach.

I have worked with a number of hospitals in Florida and Kentucky who have chosen the PSWP approach for peer review. Their philosophy is that, rather than have the medical staff avoid peer review out of fear of discovery, they would prefer a healthly peer review program that focuses on improvement even if it requires additional rework for situations resulting in formal corrective action or restriction of privileges. I agree that this is the best way to deal with a difficult legal dilemma in those states. But for most medical staffs in most states, the protection they currently enjoy far outweighs the need for the use of a PSO in peer review.

Affirmative Duty to Keep Information Confidential

The confidentiality requirement imposes an affirmative duty on the peer review committee members to keep information involving peer review to themselves. Because members of the peer review committee have such an affirmative duty, if they improperly disclose information, they may open themselves up to a potential lawsuit for "violation of a legal duty," which may be easier to prove than, for example, a defamation case. Improper disclosure of peer review information also may negate the immunity conferred by state law/HCQIA. There are a few states that impose criminal penalties (e.g., a $500 fine) for wrongful disclosure of peer review information.

A variety of state laws contain exceptions to this duty; for example, it may not apply in criminal proceedings. Consult legal counsel before disclosing peer review information outside of the peer review context.

LEGAL CONSIDERATIONS: IMPACT OF REGULATIONS AND LIABILITY ON PEER REVIEW

Fair Hearings

Any recommendation from the medical executive committee that results in an "adverse action" (e.g., restriction of privileges or membership for more than 30 days) must be addressed in accordance with the fair hearing procedures required by The Joint Commission and outlined in the medical staff bylaws and rules. Physicians have the right to a hearing, known as procedural due process, which provides them with a formal mechanism by which to ensure fairness and consideration of all relevant competency information. These safeguards give the physician the opportunity to challenge the adverse action and to present his or her own position. This process must be defined in a fair hearing plan or as provisions in the medical staff bylaws. It is important to remember, however, that simply appearing before the peer review committee to answer questions is not the same as having a fair hearing.

Medical staff bylaws must be very clear as to what will trigger the right to a fair hearing. It should occur only when an action has been taken that restricts, limits, or revokes a practitioner's hospital privileges. Consult with legal counsel to be sure your medical staff understands what actions trigger a fair hearing.

The National Practitioner Data Bank

The National Practitioner Data Bank (NPDB) is a national register of physicians, dentists, and other healthcare practitioners established pursuant to the HCQIA. Its stated objective is "to improve the quality of healthcare by encouraging hospitals … to identify and discipline those who engage in unprofessional behavior; and to restrict the ability of incompetent physicians … to move from state to state without disclosure or discovery of previous medical malpractice payment and adverse action history."

Hospitals must report to the NPDB anytime they take a professional review action that adversely affects clinical privileges of a physician for a period longer than 30 days. Hospitals also must report the voluntary surrender or restriction of clinical privileges by a physician either while that physician is under investigation or in return for not conducting an investigation.

CHAPTER 3

Many hospitals do not consider it necessary to report a letter of reprimand or a requirement to take continuing education. In addition, an investigation may be defined narrowly in medical staff bylaws; thus, informally looking into a questionable incident should not be considered an investigation.

Other times, however, the situation is less clear-cut. For example, suspending a physician for failure to complete charts might or might not relate to professional incompetence or misconduct. While currently this would not be reportable, this issue has become somewhat controversial and the requirements may change in the future. Figure 3.1 presents some examples of what types of action must be reported.

3.1 Determining NPDB Reportable Actions

Action	Report
Based on an assessment of professional competence, a proctor is assigned to a physician for a period of more than 30 days. The physician must be granted approval before administering certain medical care.	Yes
Based on an assessment of professional competence, a proctor is assigned to a physician, but the proctor does not grant approval before medical care is provided by the physician.	No
As a matter of routine hospital policy, a proctor is assigned to supervise a physician's recently granted clinical privileges.	No
A physician voluntarily restricts or surrenders clinical privileges for personal reasons; professional competence or conduct is not under investigation.	No
A physician voluntarily restricts or surrenders clinical privileges; professional competence or conduct is under investigation.	Yes
A physician voluntarily restricts or surrenders clinical privileges in return for not conducting an investigation of professional competence or conduct.	Yes
A physician's application for medical staff appointment is denied based on professional competence or conduct.	Yes
A physician is denied medical staff appointment or clinical privileges because a healthcare entity has too many specialists in the physician's discipline.	No
A physician's clinical privileges are suspended for administrative reasons not related to professional competence or conduct.	No
A physician's request for clinical privileges is denied or restricted based upon assessment of clinical competence as defined by hospital.	Yes

Negligent Peer Review

The last legal issue is one that places the organization at risk rather than the physician reviewer or the peer review committee. Plaintiff attorneys have successfully promoted the concept in court that if the peer review process was flawed and did not detect or address substandard care, the hospital can be sued for corporate negligence. This is called negligent peer review and is related to a similar concept with a flawed credentialing process, negligent credentialing.

Negligent peer review can occur in two ways: knowing information and not dealing with it (e.g., a surgeon has a mortality rate three times higher than expected) or not knowing something that you should (e.g., not collecting data on indications for coronary stent placement and a patient is harmed by a cardiologist who routinely places stents in arteries with minimal occlusions).

If the court rules that the hospital was negligent in addressing either of these two issues, the hospital can be sued for corporate negligence which allows the plaintiff access to much "deeper pockets" than the medial negligence claim. While this book is focused on doing effective peer review to improve patient care, if hospitals need an additional stimulus, the plaintiffs' pursuit of the use of negligent peer review unfortunately can provide it.

Peer Review Structures: The Impact of Multi-Specialty Peer Review

Louis Sullivan, considered by some to be America's first modern architect, coined the phrase "Form follows function." Although form should follow function, function is definitely affected by form. Sports cars and SUVs are transportation vehicles, but the design, or form, of each affects how it functions in terms of seating and cargo capacity, not to mention speed. This chapter discusses the pros and cons of the common peer review structures used currently and how these structures (i.e., "form") relate to performance improvement-focused peer review (i.e., "function").

There is no one "right" structure for peer review. Although this may be distressing for those who simply want to do the minimum necessary to meet Joint Commission and other standards, it is a plus for those who want to do effective peer review while meeting the needs of their particular medical staff culture and resources. That said, as suggested from this chapter's title and from working with medical staff over the past 10 years, preference for multi-specialty review structures is evolving, so greater emphasis will be placed on this model than in earlier editions of this book.

Why should you consider a new structure for peer review? Just as a 20-story Sullivan skyscraper was a great architectural achievement for the turn of the 20th century, it would not be able to sustain the demands for greater height and complex engineer functions required of tall buildings today. In evaluating your peer review structure, the key question is whether its current form, which may have served you well in the past, meets the more complex needs of physician performance evaluation and improvement of today and the future.

A great architect bases his design on fundamental principles. For example, Ludwig Mies van der Rohe, the designer of the steel and glass skyscrapers in the 1930s, promoted simplicity. His motto was "less is more." So what are the principles guiding the design of your peer review structure? Whatever structure you choose, make sure that it is able to support a process that minimizes bias and promotes efficiency.

CHAPTER 4

Peer Review Structures: Three Primary Functions

When designing a building, the first step is to understand functions you are trying to achieve. For example, is the building intended for commercial or residential use? An effective peer review structure must be able to accommodate three main functions:

- Physician performance evaluation
- Measurement system oversight
- Physician improvement accountability

Let's begin by exploring these further.

Physician performance evaluation

The evaluation function is the one to which many medical staff members are accustomed to through the review of individual cases. However, as was mentioned in Chapter 1, today physician performance evaluation involves more than just chart review. Now it includes looking at rate measures and compliance with rule indicators. To do this second type of evaluation effectively requires target setting to determine when a physician may have improvement opportunity. The majority of this chapter will address this function.

Measurement system oversight

In the past, the oversight of physician performance measurement by the medical staff was an afterthought—they may have done only what the quality staff told them to do. This is not the quality staff's fault but the fault of the medical staff by lack of engagement. The lack of physician leadership engagement not only causes a general ignorance of the peer review process, such as how cases are selected for review or what indicators should be measured by rates, but it also leads to a mistrust of the peer review system because there is minimal physician buy-in on how they are being measured.

With The Joint Commission standards for ongoing professional practice evaluation (OPPE) and increasing data availability through information systems and electronic medical records, the oversight of this function takes on even greater importance. It also ensures that the non-specialty areas of the general competencies are appropriately measured using a common target for evaluation across all specialties. To create an evaluation process that focuses on physician improvement, the medical staff must establish an active oversight of physician measurement with clearly assigned responsibilities.

PEER REVIEW STRUCTURES: THE IMPACT OF MULTI-SPECIALTY PEER REVIEW

There's another aspect of measurement system oversight that I have identified over the past few years regarding receiving data from other medical staff committees. Surprisingly, when asked about whether the medical staff gets data from contracted groups that do their own peer review, such as radiology or anesthesiology, the answer has often been that they've been trying but haven't been able to get the data or because it's a contracted group they did not see that as a medical staff responsibility. Part of the measurement system oversight is to be sure that all groups that are measuring physician performance are accountable and provide information to the medical staff to ensure the processes occurring in the evaluation are appropriate.

Physician improvement accountability

As the evaluation of physician performance moves from OPPE to focused professional practice evaluation (FPPE), individual physician leaders, such as department chairs, are often assigned responsibilities to either evaluate data or design performance improvement plans. Unfortunately, the accountability of these individuals is often not clear. When this occurs, it is not uncommon to have physician improvement opportunities go unevaluated or unaddressed. Defining clearly in the peer review structure who is accountable to whom and creating mechanisms to ensure accountability is the key to actually improving performance, as opposed to simply evaluating care.

CRITICAL RESPONSIBILITIES FOR EFFECTIVE OVERSIGHT OF THE PEER REVIEW PROCESS

- ❏ Standardize and coordinate the case review process to ensure reliability
- ❏ Ensure consistent interpretation of physician performance data
- ❏ Select relevant physician measures for all performance dimensions or general competencies
- ❏ Ensure that data is systematically collected and analyzed
- ❏ Ensure that identified performance improvement opportunities are addressed
- ❏ Ensure availability of physician performance data for feedback and reappointment
- ❏ Prioritize the use of resources for measuring physician performance

Chapter 4

Goals for Peer Review Structure Design

There are three important goals the effective peer review structure should try to achieve: minimize bias, increase reliability, and improve efficiency. In other words, be fair, be consistent, and don't waste physician or staff time. Let's look at how each of these may affect the peer review model options.

Minimize bias

As discussed in Chapter 2, the two types of bias most strongly affecting peer review structures are individual and group bias. Individual bias is when a given individual's relationships or values may affect the evaluation. Individual bias can be minimized when the individual's decisions are vetted by a group or at least one other individual.

Group bias is when an entire group's values or relationships may affect the evaluation. Professional bias (e.g., physicians may view things differently than nurses) and specialty bias (e.g., internists may view things differently than surgeons) are common types of group bias that may be seen in peer review. Group biases can be minimized by carefully defining the composition of a peer review committee.

Increase reliability

A reliable peer review process is one that produces consistent results. If one reviewer determines that care is appropriate, would the majority of other reviewers agree most of the time? Similarly, if the peer review committee determines that care was inappropriate, would the same committee, with different members, reach the same conclusion a year later? For a process that is reliable, the answer to both questions should be yes.

Reliability is adversely affected if a larger number of reviewers and committees perform reviews. It also is affected by how effective medical staff oversight is. For example, does the oversight function extend to matters such as ensuring the adequacy of reviewer and committee training?

For these reasons, examining the oversight structure, as well as the number and complexity of the committees to be overseen, is important. Remember, a consistent process is not only perceived to be fairer—it is fairer.

PEER REVIEW STRUCTURES: THE IMPACT OF MULTI-SPECIALTY PEER REVIEW

Improve efficiency

Efficiency means achieving a result using the minimum amount of resources. In peer review, the primary resource is time: physician time and support staff time. The three main factors that affect time are the types of measures used to evaluate physician performance (discussed in Chapter 5), the procedures used in the evaluation process, and the number of committees and individuals involved.

Having multiple departmental peer review committees means more physician time is spent in peer review meetings, not to mention the time that administrative support staff spend organizing the meetings and preparing the documents. The hours quickly add up. Imagine a hospital with 10 departmental monthly peer review committee meetings: If each committee has five physicians, and the meetings last an average of 1.5 hours, meetings take 900 physician-hours annually. If another five hours of staff time is spent to prepare and support each meeting, 600 more hours per year are invested in the peer review system—and that doesn't even account for the time the quality department personnel spend actually vetting cases and screening them for the physicians.

Using many peer review committees is also less efficient for individual physicians and staff. Physicians will be less familiar, hence less efficient, with the case review process if they do it infrequently, and staff will be less efficient if they have to track down many different physicians to get the reviews done.

Basic Peer Review Models

You can achieve each of the above goals of effective peer review using a variety of structural models. The key question is which model will best reinforce your peer review cultural values while promoting efficient use of physician and staff time within the context of your hospital and medical staff organizational structure. The goal of this chapter is to help you decide if you have the right model for your peer review program today.

There are two basic models that drive peer review:

- Department or specialty-based (for the purpose of this chapter we will refer to this as specialty-based)

- Multi-specialty-based

CHAPTER 4

The underlying premise for each model is based on a medical staff's definition of a peer. As mentioned in Chapter 1, a peer may be restricted to a physician in the specialty of the physician being evaluated or may have a broader definition of a physician with the appropriate expertise for the specific issue under evaluation. The first definition would likely lead to a peer review structure based in departments or specialties. The second definition provides the option of multi-specialty peer review. However, as will be discussed below, a medical staff may sometimes mix elements from each of these two models.

Now let's look at how the structures generally created from these two basic models try to accomplish the three peer review goals previously discussed.

Specialty-based peer review models

The specialty-based peer review model is the most commonly used because it is the traditional model. It derives in part from the university setting, where peer review and mortality and morbidity (M&M) conferences were, in the past, often combined. It was also driven by The Joint Commission's approach to peer review that asked every department to develop at least two indicators. This emphasized to the medical staff that peer review was primarily a department-based function.

There are two main ways specialty-based peer review can be structured:

- Department chair model
- Department committee model

Department chair model

This model is typically found in academic hospitals where the appointed department chair reviews all quality-of-care issues, interacts directly with the physician involved, and comes to a conclusion without input from others. It is, in effect, a committee of one. This model also applies to community hospitals where the elected department chair is assigned this responsibility. A variation on this model seen in nonacademic settings is where the department chair is designated as the initial reviewer for all cases but, if there is an issue, the case is discussed by a committee.

This model is simple, and in keeping with the saying that a dictatorship is the most efficient form of government, a single individual often makes more efficient decisions than a committee. It has significant drawbacks, however, in terms of individual and specialty bias. Being the sole determiner of a physician's performance can lead to the perception—if not the reality—of individual bias. Although some chairs might abuse this authority, it typically results in the underscoring of cases. For example, an academic chair may feel pressured to ignore poor care because the physician under review is an academic or research superstar. In a community setting, the elected chair may only serve for a year or two and does not want to make waves.

Inter-reliability issues are less of a concern where department chairs are appointed and have long tenure. However, inter-reliability can be a concern in community hospitals where the elected chair position turns over frequently.

Department committee model

In this model, a clinical department selects a subset of its members (usually between five and 10) to meet at prescribed times (usually monthly) to perform case reviews. Sometimes this group is also used for other departmental activities such as credentialing or performance improvement projects. Cases identified for review usually are assigned to a reviewer prior to the meeting. The committee meets to discuss the relevant charts and other materials and determines whether care was appropriate. Departmental peer review committees also may determine the indicators to be used, typically by reviewing last year's list and making minor changes.

The role of the department chair in this model may vary. In some organizations, the department chair may be the committee chair or a committee member. In others, the department chair is only involved in the improvement opportunities once the committee makes its decision.

This model can have significant issues related to bias, reliability, and efficiency. Indeed, although this model is widely used, its failure is the most common reason that The Greeley Company has been asked to help medical staffs redesign their peer review process.

In relation to bias, a departmental peer review committee certainly reduces the individual bias concern present in the department chair model, especially if the department chair is not on the committee. However, it is strongly affected by specialty-group bias and, because of the group process it uses, often magnifies that bias. In addition, reliability problems stem from the multiplicity of reviewers and the potential variability in how different departments perform the process. Regarding efficiency, it is the least efficient model because of the number of department and section committees often involved. For example, it is not uncommon in this model to find departments with only three members having their own committee. It is also inefficient in how it handles cases with multiple different specialists involved in the care. Typically, one department sends the case to the other department for review or it may be discussed in both departments simultaneously. For example, a case of perioperative myocardial infarction would be discussed at both the surgery and anesthesiology committees. Ironically, despite the fact the surgeon and the anesthesiologist provided care together in the same room, because of committee structure, the discussion on how to improve that care must occur in separate rooms.

Multi-specialty peer review models

Today, hospitalized patients are sicker and have more complex needs than in the past, and many medical staffs now recognize that patient care must be a collaborative effort. As a result, there has been a movement toward creating multi-specialty committees to perform peer review.

There is a need to make a distinction between two terms that are sometimes confused: multi-specialty and multidisciplinary. Multi-specialty means voting committee members are physicians from various specialties. Multidisciplinary means that voting members are from different disciplines (e.g., physician, nurse, physical therapist). As will be discussed later in this chapter, while I have found a few non-voting representatives from other disciplines can reduce professional bias, I do not advocate multidisciplinary peer review.

There are two main ways multi-specialty-based peer review can be structured:

- The single, central multi-specialty committee
- The multiple multi-specialty committees

The single, central multi-specialty peer review committee model

This is the most common model that medical staffs are adopting. In this model, a single, multi-specialty peer review committee performs all case reviews and performs the oversight functions related to other measures of physician performance. Typically, the committee is composed of seven to nine physicians from different specialties or departments. The number of members can be greater but the goal is not to have representation from every specialty. It is to create a cadre of dedicated, clinically credible, and respected peer reviewers who are well trained in the peer review process. Thus, the terms of appointment tend to be longer (e.g., in the three- to five-year range), with a staggering of the terms to provide more continuity of the process.

Peer review committee members act as the initial physician reviewers, but if additional clinical expertise is needed, the committee can request assistance from any specialist on the medical staff who the committee thinks would be most appropriate. All determinations of appropriateness of care, however, are made by the committee. Another advantage is that, as a single, centralized committee, it can look at all physicians involved in the care and their interactions in a single review. Additionally, many physicians enjoy the cross-disciplinary dialogue and learning, which increases participation.

In this model, the peer review committee only makes recommendations regarding improvement strategies. The department chair is responsible for working with the physician under review on the actual improvement approach. This separates the evaluation portion of the peer review process from the action or implementation portion. This distinction is important because medical staff bylaws usually state that the elected medical staff leaders, including the department chairs and the officers of the medical executive committee (MEC), must take action. Implementing this model does not change that.

This model has many advantages over the specialty-based models because it:

- Minimizes bias: Because this model is multi-specialty, there is less individual and specialty bias. It brings multiple perspectives to the table during the evaluation process instead of adding them after the fact via a second department review or appeal to an oversight committee.

- Increases reliability: With a single, centralized committee, there are fewer reviewers to train, and as they work together over time, they will normalize the evaluation process and increase reliability. It also removes the issue of variability because there is only one committee.

- Improves efficiency: It is more efficient for staff because it has the fewest committees to support and it eliminates the need for establishing a separate oversight committee. It also reduces the number of physician participants required for peer review. In an age with declining physician involvement in medical staff functions, this is an attractive feature of this model. Also, because the committee reports directly to the MEC, it consolidates the quality reporting processes.

One concern often raised about this model is that, with fewer physicians doing peer review, those physicians would be doing more work and would quickly become overloaded. However, this committee is also responsible for the oversight of performance measures. Once it is educated on the proper use of rate and rule indicators, it can limit physician chart review to only those cases that are of a serious or complex nature resulting in a decrease in the amount of time required for physician chart review.

The major criticism of this model is the potential lack of appropriate specialty expertise or the view that only one member of a specialty will perform all initial reviews for that specialty. However, as discussed earlier, many cases identified for peer review raise only the question of general medical care, which is easily evaluated by any physician on the peer review committee. In fact, many of these committees assign initial physician review of cases by rotation rather than by specialty. Then, if the initial reviewer needs additional specialty expertise, the committee can obtain it on an ad hoc basis.

A more minor concern sometimes raised is that with fewer physicians involved in the peer review process, those not involved lose the opportunity to learn from the clinical activity of others. However, education is the role of the M&M conference, not of peer review. The peer review system should be active in identifying potential cases for M&M discussions.

Although this model was originally thought to be best-suited for smaller hospitals, I have seen a significant trend of medium-size hospitals (300–400 beds) finding this model effective for that setting. Surprisingly, a number of large tertiary-care academic medical centers have also recently and successfully implemented this model by maintaining strong departmental M&Ms separate from peer review and moving to rate and rule indicators to limit the number of cases requiring physician review.

The multiple multi-specialty peer review committees model

Some organizations are attracted to the concept of multi-specialty review but are concerned that the complexity of their services may make it too burdensome for a single committee, or they wish to enhance care collaboration in a more-focused manner. This has led some medical staffs to adopt the multiple multi-specialty committees model. Such peer review committees have multi-specialty representation but may be organized by service lines (e.g., cardiovascular, maternal/child, trauma), diseases (e.g., respiratory), units (e.g., intensive care, emergency services), or a combination of those categories. It also may result from combining many small departments into a larger committee (e.g., all medical specialties and subspecialties meet as a single committee).

What are the downsides? If there are too many of these committees (e.g., more than four or five), this approach still requires substantial staff support and oversight to ensure reliability; thus, efficiency and reliability may suffer. Also, to have truly multi-specialty committees, some hospital-based departments (e.g., emergency medicine and anesthesiology) will need to participate in several committees like a cardiovascular, maternal/child, or respiratory diseases peer review committee.

A variation of this model that some medical staffs have tried is to consolidate multiple committees in the same general specialty (e.g., a single surgical peer review committee for all surgery departments and subspecialties). Although superficially this may appear to be multi-specialty, it is actually just a more-efficient version of the specialty-based peer review committee model since the "specialties" involved come from the same root specialty. It can become more truly multi-specialty if physicians from other root specialties are added to each committee (e.g., an emergency medicine physician is appointed to the surgery committee).

Combined department committees and multi-specialty committee model

Some medical staffs have been reluctant to abandon department committees but want to have a better forum to address cases involving multiple departments and ensure consistency among the committees. To that end, they have established a multi-specialty oversight committee that can review cases involving more than one physician. Of course, this is not highly efficient, but it can be an initial step in moving toward a multi-specialty review committee in the face of strong department-based culture.

Who Should Oversee Peer Review?

Regardless of the model, peer review requires active oversight to ensure it is running as intended. Depending on the model, several options are available. The key principle is that if the model has more than two committees, some form of oversight committee is typically needed.

In the department-based models, the individual committees may report directly to the MEC or to a medical staff quality committee. Unless a hospital is small, the MEC tends not to have the time to provide effective oversight, and using a separate committee that reports to the MEC is a better approach. This committee may have varying degrees of responsibility ranging from simply being a forum for reporting to reviewing cases that cross departmental lines.

The single multi-specialty committee handles the oversight functions and typically reports directly to the MEC just like the credentials committee. If there are more than two or three multi-specialty committees, some type of oversight committee is needed to ensure consistency and deal with medical staffwide issues. This committee is often composed of the chairs of each of the multi-specialty committees, which would then report to the MEC.

Selecting the Right Model

How do you decide which model is best for your medical staff? Albert Einstein once said, "All things should be as simple as possible, but no simpler." In other words, there is a polarity between simplicity and necessary complexity. And as our stated goal is to have an unbiased, reliable, and efficient process (i.e., function), any structure (i.e., form) must enhance—or at a minimum, not detract from—that goal. In addition to bias, reliability, and efficiency, consider how much cultural change would be needed before your medical staff would accept a new model. As an aid, Figure 4.1 briefly summarizes the effect of each model on reliability, bias, and efficiency.

What is the current trend? There is no question that many medical staffs are moving to some form of multi-specialty peer review. As mentioned at the beginning of this chapter, I have a bias in favor of this approach because we have seen the positive effects it has on a medical staff's ability to create a performance improvement–focused culture for peer review. In addition to its advantages in relation to the three basic functions, the most compelling aspect is the inter-specialty dialogue and learning that occurs. As a result, physician participation in the committees is usually very high because the committee members feel that the time spent is worthwhile.

4.1 Impact of Peer Review Evaluation Models

	Minimize personal bias	Minimize specialty bias	Reliability	Efficiency	Total points	Culture change
Department chair (academic)	Poor (0)	Poor (0)	Fair (1)	Good (2)	3	Minimal
Department chair (elected)	Poor (0)	Poor (0)	Fair (1)	Fair (1)	2	Minimal
Department committees	Fair (1)	Poor (0)	Poor (0)	Poor (0)	1	Minimal
Department committees with multi-specialty oversight committee	Fair (1)	Fair (1)	Fair (1)	Poor (0)	3	Moderate
Multiple multi-specialty committees	Good (2)	Good (2)	Good (2)	Fair (1)	7	Moderate-High
Single multi-specialty committee	Good (2)	Good (2)	Good (2)	Good (2)	8	High

Key:
Poor: 0 points
Fair: 1 point
Good: 2 points

PEER REVIEW STRUCTURES: THE IMPACT OF MULTI-SPECIALTY PEER REVIEW

Multidisciplinary Membership and Participation in Peer Review

Deciding whether to have nonphysicians, such as nurses, participate in peer review is a culture issue (although it is also wise to consult with your legal counsel to make sure that having nonphysicians participate in peer review does not jeopardize any peer review legal protections). Many medical staffs allow the quality management support staffs who perform the initial case screening to be present and to add to the discussion. Indeed, having a nursing or a risk management perspective can add value as well. Some medical staffs even have a lay board member present.

The main question when making the decision about who to include in peer review is whether the presence of nonphysicians would inhibit candid discussion. Although that is often cited as the reason for preventing nonphysician participation, in many instances it has the opposite effect: When no one else is in the room, physicians sometimes excuse activities that other disciplines might question. Thus, allowing nonphysician participation is a way to reduce professional bias. Another benefit of nonphysician participation is linkage to other disciplines when system or process issues are identified. A third benefit is that it increases credibility and trust in the peer review process by the rest of the organization.

For multidisciplinary participation to work well, three criteria must be met. First, only physicians should be permitted to vote on matters of physician performance. Second, participation is a privilege granted by the medical staff. It is based on trust that the participant will maintain confidentiality and the independence of the process from management. Any breach of that trust would result in loss of participation. Third, the number of nonphysicians should be limited—physician discussion may become inhibited if they sense that they are being observed. If these criteria can be met, I would encourage nonphysician participation in peer review.

Physician Behavior: Who Should Handle It?

A common question is whether physician behavior issues (i.e., so-called disruptive behaviors) should be handled by the peer review committee or by some other method. While these behaviors fall under the core competency of professionalism, handling them at a peer review committee can be both time-consuming and divert from the main focus of the committee, which is to improve patient care.

Medical staffs that handle these issues through a separate mechanism do a better job of addressing these issues. Typical approaches are through a separate physician wellness committee or through direct involvement by medical staff leaders.

CHOOSING A NAME FOR YOUR COMMITTEE

If you decide to redesign your committee structure, it will need a new name before it is ready to go. When it comes to naming your medical staff quality committee, you can choose from a number of possibilities. Sometimes the old name has baggage, so something different is needed. Some medical staffs want to declare a new beginning for peer review and choose a name that announces this intent. Others want to be sure the committee's purpose is clear from its title. Below are some of the names I have seen used over the past few years:

- MSQC: Medical Staff Quality Committee
- MSQOC: Medical Staff Quality Oversight Committee
- PEC: Physician Excellence Committee
- PEC: Practitioner Evaluation Committee
- PIC: Physician Improvement Committee
- PPC: Physician Performance Committee
- PPIC: Physician Performance Improvement Committee
- PPC: Professional Practice Committee
- PPEC: Professional Practice Excellence Committee
- PPEC: Professional Practice Evaluation Committee
- PIC: Professional Improvement Committee
- PRC: Peer Review Committee

5. Measuring Physician Performance: What to Measure and How to Do It Fairly

When asked how they perform peer review, physicians often conjure up images of poring over a stack of charts in the back of the medical records office or sitting in a committee meeting trying to decide whether a patient outcome can be truly attributed to a specific physician's performance. However, if asked how they measure physician performance, their responses broaden to include other means of evaluation, especially if they recognize that there are multiple aspects of physician performance, as discussed in Chapter 1.

What physicians often don't realize is that how to perform peer review and how to measure physician performance are different versions of the same question. As noted at the beginning of this book, peer review is the evaluation of an individual physician's professional performance by other physicians. Although case review is one tool to evaluate physician performance, many tools are available today to help with this task.

A carpenter starting to build a cabinet will make sure that he or she has all the right tools in his or her tool belt before beginning. Likewise, to measure physician performance, you must first take stock of your performance measurement tool belt and be sure you understand how to use each tool.

What Is a Physician Performance Indicator?

Performance measures, also called indicators, do more than provide data: They indicate how something is actually performing. For example, the speedometer indicates how fast a car is going, and although a driver might have a general idea of speed from his or her own driving experience, using a speedometer is more objective. Similarly, physicians may have a good sense of another physician's performance if they have worked with that physician, but actually defining performance indicators provides a more objective way for physicians to evaluate each other. Such indicators are particularly important because not all physicians will have had the opportunity to work with, or observe the work of, the physician under review.

Indicator Validity: Selecting Physician-Driven Measures

The most common question asked by physicians regarding physician performance data is, "Does this data really measure physician performance?" This question is particularly important when data is being applied to individual physicians in an ongoing professional practice evaluation (OPPE). The issue that is being raised is whether the data is valid. Unless physicians agree to the data's validity, they will be unwilling to use it to improve their performance.

The definition of validity is that "a measure measures what is purported to measure." For physician performance data, this means that somehow you can show that the data is indeed driven by actions that are in the control of the physician. If variation in data is due to hospital systems or processes—rather than physician performance—the indicator is not valid to use for OPPE.

For example, the ordering of the appropriate antibiotic for pneumonia patients is a valid physician performance indicator since only physicians can write orders. However, patient falls are typically not a valid physician performance indicator because most of the causes are outside the physician's control.

As we move forward to further discuss indicators in this chapter and later chapters, keep in mind that the first question to answer is whether what is being proposed as a physician performance measure is physician-driven. If not, then keep it off the peer review indicator list.

What Are You Required to Measure?

In today's regulatory-driven environment, there is a tendency to start with the question, "What are we required to measure?" and, unfortunately, end there as well. The question you should start with is, "What is useful to measure regarding physician competency?" and then make sure the regulatory requirements are satisfied. If you answer the usefulness question honestly, you will almost always cover the requirements.

Interestingly, there are no specifically required indicators for physician peer review. While there are many traditional indicators used in peer review, these are based on the Centers for Medicare & Medicaid Services (CMS) and Joint Commission requirements that the hospital monitor and evaluate certain functions (e.g., blood use, operative procedures) and conditions (e.g., mortality, complications). There also is required data for hospitals to collect regarding important processes, such as core measures.

MEASURING PHYSICIAN PERFORMANCE: WHAT TO MEASURE AND HOW TO DO IT FAIRLY

While physicians may have a role in many of these measures, the regulations do not define what indicators must be used on a physician-specific level. Even with the adoption of the six core competences for OPPE, The Joint Commission does not define what indicators are to be measured for each competency. Thus, there is a great deal of flexibility in physician performance measurement. Instead of embracing this flexibility, organizations often struggle to determine the best physician performance measures for their individual organization. It is important to spend the time and effort to determine which measures are relevant to your physicians.

To start, classify your physician performance indicators by asking two questions: what to measure and how to measure it. The answers to the first question are based on the classic Donabedian model of assessing quality of care. The answers to the second question are based on The Greeley Company's three methods of analyzing performance: chart review, rule compliance, and rate of a particular occurrence.

What to Measure: Structure, Process, and Outcome

According to the classic Donabedian triangle[1] (see Figure 5.1), you can assess the quality of medical care by looking at information about structure, process, or outcome. The idea is that good structure increases the likelihood of good process and that good process increases the likelihood of good outcome. But knowing exactly what it is about structure, process, or outcome that is actually related to quality is no easy task, as we will discuss next.

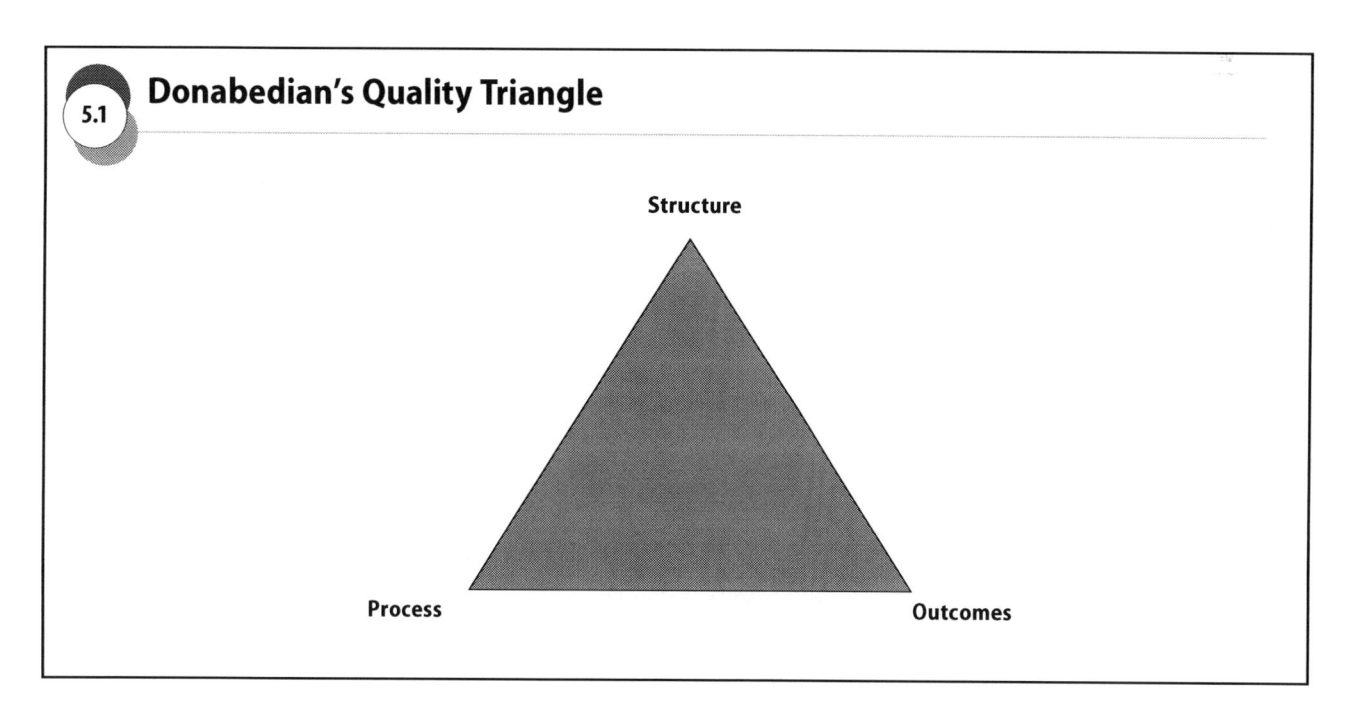

Figure 5.1 Donabedian's Quality Triangle

(Triangle with vertices labeled: Structure (top), Process (bottom left), Outcomes (bottom right))

Structure indicators

Structure indicators relate the attributes of the setting in which care occurs (e.g., the facilities, equipment, or services provided by a hospital) or of an individual providing the care (e.g., the board-certification status of the physician) to some desirable result. Structure indicators are yes or no questions: Does the particular attribute we are looking for exist or not?

Consider the following question: Which hospital has the best chance of preserving an acute myocardial infarction (AMI) patient's myocardium: Hospital A, which offers only thrombolytic therapy, or Hospital B, which offers both thrombolytic therapy and interventional cardiac procedures? We can answer this question without even knowing how fast or how well the cardiac intervention could be performed. That's because we know that not all AMI patients qualify for thrombolytics and that studies have shown that interventions such as angioplasty and placing intra-arterial stents will preserve myocardium. Thus, because Hospital B has a particular capability, or structure, an AMI patient treated there is more likely to have a better outcome.

Structure indicator data are generally easier to obtain than process or outcomes. However, structure measures do not change rapidly. For example, a physician board-certification status does not change every quarter or six months. Therefore, use of structure measures to evaluate physician performance is generally relegated to the initial and biennial credentialing cycle but not in OPPE.

Process indicators

Process refers to how the physician delivers care. For example, a good process indicator for interventional cardiology available at Hospital B would be the time it takes to begin the catheterization procedure or the so-called "door-to-wire" time. Why? Because clinical studies show that the more quickly this procedure is performed, the better the quality of care as defined by myocardial preservation. And although performing a process well does not guarantee good quality, it is more closely associated with quality than simply meeting a structure indicator.

But why measure process and not just measure the outcome? One reason is that measuring a process is often easier because it occurs in the present and at the hospital. An outcome, on the other hand, may occur at some distant time or place. For example, because of short hospital stays, inpatient surgical wound infections often are not detected until after patients are discharged. Obtaining this outcome data from each surgeon's office would be quite difficult. However, studies show that timely preoperative prophylactic antibiotics reduce infection, so measuring the performance of the process of giving timely prophylactic antibiotics gives a good indication of the likelihood of fewer infections.

MEASURING PHYSICIAN PERFORMANCE: WHAT TO MEASURE AND HOW TO DO IT FAIRLY

Unfortunately, as with structure indicators, it is easy to measure all kinds of processes, and hospitals sometimes do so just to show they have data on quality. But there should be reasonable evidence of a process-outcome relationship before measuring a process—simply assuming the connection is not enough. Good process indicators measure processes that link to the desired outcome.

Outcome indicators

Outcome refers to what actually happens to the patient. Outcome indicators ask, "Did we really improve health? Did we heal? Did we avoid harm?" Returning again to Hospital B, the bottom line is the mortality and complication rates for the invasive cardiac procedures. It doesn't matter how quickly they're done if they aren't done well. Although outcome indicators often are discussed in terms of defined clinical outcomes, as in the preceding example, efficient resource use, such as length of stay, is also a measurable outcome.

The purpose for measuring outcomes is to find ways to improve them. Many outcome indicators today are being defined by medical specialties, payers, regulators, the government, and consumers so that physicians will have data they can use to improve their performance. Ironically, the best way to improve performance (i.e., the outcome) is to improve the process that produced the outcome. Therefore, although improving outcomes is the end goal, these outcomes must be reasonably linked to processes that can be understood and actually be improved.

For example, when Medicare provided hospitals with overall inpatient risk-adjusted mortality data in the late 1980s, most hospitals did not know what to do with it. There was no clear link between general mortality and specific clinical processes (other than the consistent flaws in medical record coding). However, once data was provided on disease-specific mortality, such as AMI or coronary bypass surgery, hospitals and doctors could examine how care was delivered (i.e., the process) and find ways to improve it.

The best rule to apply when selecting outcome or process measures is to be sure that the process is linked to a known outcome that you want to improve and that the outcome is linked to a known process. That way, the physician knows what to improve. Sometimes you may wish to measure both process and outcome on the same performance area because even though it may be easy to measure just the outcome, intervention can occur earlier if you also measure the process.

CHAPTER 5

How to Measure Physicians Fairly: Review, Rate, and Rule Indicators

Over the past 15 years, The Greeley Company has developed and implemented a way to describe physician performance measurement tools that reduces the focus and, subsequently, the time physicians spend on chart review while still providing accurate information on physician performance. It shifts the peer review process away from reviewing individual cases to reviewing more aggregate data. Most medical staffs have found that this approach works, although as with most things, some variance from this approach may be needed from time to time.

Physician performance indicators can be divided into three categories: review, rule, and rate indicators. Using these indicator categories can help the medical staff and administrative support personnel to fairly and efficiently evaluate and act upon issues that arise in the peer review process. These categories are based on three principles:

- Fairness: Is the potential physician performance issue most fairly evaluated as an individual event or as a performance pattern or trend?

- Focus: For individual events, does the complexity of the potential physician care issue require direct physician evaluation of the event?

- Feedback: For patterns and trends, is it more effective for performance improvement to make the physician aware of the occurrence for each event or only when sufficient data has been collected to determine whether a pattern is present?

Now let's explore how these principles can help you select the right approach for physician performance indicators.

Review indicators

Review indicators, sometimes called review criteria or triggers, identify situations in which individual charts or circumstances must be reviewed in detail by an appropriate physician—that is, by traditional peer review. The reason for the review is to determine the effectiveness and appropriateness of the care provided by the physician.

Generally, a review indicator describes a relatively broad significant adverse patient outcome (e.g., mortality, readmission, complication) or significant process (delay in treatment) that may or may not relate

MEASURING PHYSICIAN PERFORMANCE: WHAT TO MEASURE AND HOW TO DO IT FAIRLY

to physician performance. It should flag a case for detailed chart analysis when the actual (or potential) outcome for the patient is serious and too complex to be understood by measuring how frequently such outcomes occur. Usually there is an attempt to determine the cause, effect, and severity of the outcome for the patient, as well as any possible physician "failure mode," such as an error in judgment, knowledge, or skill.

A review indicator is more effective when it is more clearly spelled out, such as "unanticipated mortality," "readmission within 48 hours," or "significant post-procedure complications" (e.g., stroke, AMI, cardio-respiratory arrest). As will be discussed in Chapter 6, this allows for more effective pre-physician case screening by quality staff, which can eliminate unnecessary physician reviews.

Review indicators require specific feedback on an event-by-event basis. This process will be discussed in detail in Chapter 6 but, at a minimum, requires an opportunity for physician response and formal communication regarding the determination of the event and any improvement opportunities. The number of cases determined to have physician improvement opportunities should be tracked and a threshold target set over a period of time so that if a physician exceeds that number, it will automatically trigger a follow-up focus study (see Chapter 9 for more information).

While case review is still an important tool, the bias of this book is to help medical staff limit their use of case review to only when needed. One reason for this is review indicator case identification can be biased against high-volume providers. This is particularly true if review indicators are used for commonly expected complications that occur even in the best of care. When this happens there are usually two results: physician time is wasted with unnecessary reviews that are always rated "care appropriate–known complication" and the committee may infer a busy physician's care is below expectations. For example, Dr. Able had five complications and Dr. Mal had three, but Dr. Able treated five times as many patients as Dr. Mal. Rate indicators, discussed later in the chapter, help overcome this bias.

So how do the three principles apply to review indicators?

- Fairness: Due to the seriousness/complexity of the issues, it is only fair to have another physician review the medical record directly to determine whether the physician's rationale and actions were appropriate and effective. However, if applied to routine, expected events, review indicators may be biased against high-volume providers.

- Focus: Since review indicators require direct chart review by a physician and often extensive committee discussion, they are the most labor-intensive indicators.

- Feedback: Review indicators provide very specific feedback and often dialogue between the committee and the physician under review. However, depending on the timeliness of case identification and reviewer and committee determinations, the timeliness of the feedback can be quite variable.

Rule indicators

Rule indicators are based on the rules, standards, or generally recognized professional guidelines for the practice of medicine, and if such rules are not followed, the resulting noncompliance is unlikely to cause a patient harm. This does not mean that every rule indicator must be an official "rule" in the medical staff bylaws or rules and regulations although that is certainly a source of rule indicators. Medical staff–approved policies and practice guidelines are often used as rule indicators. Ideally, physicians should always comply with these rules, and rare or isolated deviations from these rules usually represent only minor problems.

Rule indicators generally measure a process rather than an outcome because rules typically describe a policy or procedure to be followed. Rule indicators may relate to all physician core competencies. For example, a professionalism rule indicator could be that all physicians must complete their medical records on time; a medical knowledge rule indicator could be compliance with blood transfusion criteria. The most useful rule indicators measure processes for which there is some degree of noncompliance either among the medical staff in general or with some individual physicians. Creating rule indicators for which there is already 100% compliance is not very helpful for identifying and improving physician performance.

The physician must be informed of every instance of noncompliance, no matter how many other times he or she is compliant. Those who routinely fail to comply will quickly become apparent because most physicians will be fully compliant or will have only rare incidents of noncompliance.

The medical staff should establish a target for the number of violations of a particular rule that would be considered excessive and communicate that number, in advance, to all medical staff members (see Chapter 7 for more information). Remember, setting clear expectations is an important layer in the performance pyramid discussed in Chapter 4.

The key to using rule indicators effectively is to select issues where the information can be obtained relatively objectively by nonphysicians and do not require physician chart review. Typically, when rule indicator noncompliance is identified, an automatic educational letter is sent directly to the physician

MEASURING PHYSICIAN PERFORMANCE: WHAT TO MEASURE AND HOW TO DO IT FAIRLY

by administrative support personnel, with no further action taken at that time. (See Figure 5.2 for a sample letter.) If the rule is clinical, the medical basis for the rule is attached to the notice. The letter typically does not go into the physician's quality file but the number of letters is tracked. Once that number exceeds a medical staff target, then the committee will discuss the issue.

Often raised are the questions "Aren't rule indicators unfair because they don't take into account the volume of activity for each physician?" and "Should these rules be measured as rates?" Rule indicators should be used when you don't want a physician's volume of work to be an excuse for failing to achieve high-reliability compliance. Being so busy you either don't have time to comply or forget to comply is not an acceptable practice.

For example, if a busy pilot decided there wasn't time to complete the preflight checklist because he or she had to get to the next destination, a review of the pilot's checklist completion rate would reveal noncompliance with established protocol. Similarly, many medical staffs look at late starts in the operating room as a rule indicator rather than a rate indicator because often the reason for missing scheduled start times is that the surgeon is too busy at other facilities.

So how do the three principles apply to rule indicators?

- Fairness: Rule indicators are designed to remind the physician of important policies or practices that may have been overlooked by a simple lapse or lack of understanding. Once the medical staff sets the rule indicators to be measured, all physicians are treated the same.

- Focus: Since rule indicators do not require physician chart review for each instance, they provide a more efficient use of physician reviewer and committee time.

- Feedback: Rule indicators provide a mechanism for giving physicians timely feedback when a rule is violated with the hope that the physician will self-correct prior to a trend developing.

The box on page 72 examines how to properly use a rule indicator, and Figure 5.2 is a sample letter to send physicians.

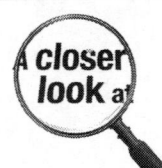

A closer look at: How to Use a Rule Indicator

Rule: No transfusion of red blood cells when hemoglobin is greater than 8 grams unless there is active bleeding or when the patient is otherwise medically unstable.

On occasion, any physician may use the "medically unstable" criterion to justify a transfusion beyond what is typically seen. If this only happens once or twice a year, an exchange of letters debating the specifics of an individual case or discussing the issue at a committee meeting is a waste of time. The physician should simply be notified of his or her violations and reminded of the rule itself. The underlying assumption of this communication is the expectation that the physician will comply with the rule going forward.

If a physician truly believed the patient was medically unstable and required transfusion, there still would be no need for response as a single violation has no effect on the overall evaluation of the physician's performance. Perhaps it was merely a documentation issue that the physician can address. However, if noncompliance with this rule exceeds the acceptable target, then the committee must begin a dialogue with the physician. Again, the focus is not on fault; rather, the first question should be, "Why do you think that your practice appears to be different from other physicians on our staff?"

What if the physician felt the rule does not apply to his or her patient population? For example, nephrologists routinely transfuse chronic dialysis patients at 9 grams of hemoglobin rather than 8. Ideally there should have been an earlier discussion between the medical staff quality committee and the specialist when the rule was first proposed and distributed for comment prior to implementation. But perhaps the newly trained nephrologist has just joined the medical staff. Identifying this nephrologist as an outlier early on allows the medical staff to consider whether to revise this particular rule indicator, which would improve its physician performance evaluation process.

MEASURING PHYSICIAN PERFORMANCE: WHAT TO MEASURE AND HOW TO DO IT FAIRLY

5.2 Sample Rule Indicator Letter

Dear Doctor _____,

The medical staff has selected a number of performance screening indicators designated as general rule indicators. These indicators represent the medical staff general rules, standards, or recognized accepted practices of medicine where individual variation does not directly cause adverse patient outcomes. Ideally, there should always be compliance with these indicators, although occasional justifiable deviations may occur.

The purpose of providing physicians with this feedback is to increase awareness of these rules or guidelines and improve future physician performance on a self-improvement basis. These indicators do not trigger any physician peer review for this case.

During a routine review of patient records based on these indicators, the medical record of patient _____ admitted on _____ for which you were listed as the attending/consulting physician was reviewed. If the patient assignment is incorrect, please inform the quality management office immediately so we can assign the patient to the appropriate physician. In this case, the documentation provided in the medical record did not reflect compliance with the following indicator:

_____
_____

There is no need for you to respond to this letter unless you are not the physician responsible for this patient's care. We only ask that you consider the feedback regarding this indicator in the spirit of continuous improvement and apply it to your future practice as appropriate for improving either documentation or approaches to patient care. Please consider this report confidential.

The medical staff quality improvement committee will also perform analysis for patterns of noncompliance with a given indicator over time. If any potential pattern is identified, the individual physician will be contacted for a response to assist in understanding the basis for that pattern.

If you have any questions or concerns about the specific indicator, please feel free to contact me, as the medical staff is always interested in improving our quality indicators.

We recognize that receiving and providing performance feedback is not always easy. Thank you for your cooperation with our efforts to try to create a positive approach to providing our physicians with this information.

Sincerely,

_____
Medical staff quality committee chair

Rate indicators

Rate indicators measure the number of events that have occurred compared to the number of opportunities for that event to have occurred. Thus, a rate indicator has a numerator and a denominator and can be expressed as a percentage, frequency, average, rank, or ratio. Rate indicators measure both processes and outcomes. They lend themselves easily to statistical analysis and to adjustment for severity of illness or for risk of adverse outcome.

Rate indicators ask whether the frequency of an adverse outcome or a failed process is different from established expectations. That is, they focus on the forest, whereas review indicators look at the trees, one by one. As noted earlier, case review can be biased against the high-volume physician. Rate indicators level the playing field by adjusting for volume.

Why use rate indicators? First, they are more efficient than review indicators because they do not require physician reviewers to review individual charts to obtain the data. Rather, the data is collected by hospital staff or hospital information systems for evaluation by the appropriate physician leader or committee.

Second, collecting rate data sometimes provides better information about physician performance. For example, perforations during colonoscopy happen even with the most experienced and competent gastroenterologists. If each case was examined individually, the usual result would be "care appropriate." Measuring how often a particular gastroenterologist causes a perforation (i.e., his or her rate of perforations) is much more useful. That rate can be compared with those of others performing the procedure at the hospital or with national reported rates of perforation.

So why not use only rate indicators for physician performance evaluation? One problem is that processes performed infrequently have low denominators; thus, any change in the numerator (the number of successes or failures) is exaggerated, and the data would not be statistically reliable.

For example, a procedure performed 50 times per month with 10 failures has a success rate of 80% (40/50), the same percentage if it was performed five times per month and failed once (4/5). In the first instance, however, one additional failure reduces the success rate to 78% (40/51), whereas in the second situation the rate drops to 66% (4/6). One solution to this problem is to use a longer time frame. For a procedure performed five times per month, looking at the aggregate data twice per year increases the number of data points to 60.

MEASURING PHYSICIAN PERFORMANCE: WHAT TO MEASURE AND HOW TO DO IT FAIRLY

As with rule indicators, the way to analyze rate indicators is to first set targets or use statistical variation analysis to define outliers. The next step is to find out why the physician is an outlier. This is now the beginning point for focused professional practice evaluation. Look at patient charts for more information, or simply discuss the situation with the physician. Remember, however, that with rate indicators, the peer review committee has to look at the charts of only the few physician outliers instead of those of every physician (as with review indicators). These two steps will be discussed further in Chapters 9 and 10.

Unlike review and rule indicators, where the feedback to the physician is provided for each individual event or occurrence, the feedback of rate indicator results should be done at regular, defined intervals (e.g., quarterly or semiannually). The time period chosen relates to the amount of data typically available so that any change in the rate would be timely and meaningful.

So how do the three principles apply to rate indicators?

- Fairness: For issues that occur as reasonable frequency for any physician, rate indicators adjust for volume of care provided for those outcomes.

- Focus: Since rate indicators do not require physician chart review for each instance, they provide a more efficient use of physician reviewer and committee time.

- Feedback: Unless dealing with very high volume, rate indicators to gather the number of numerator and denominator events will require a longer time frame to interpret (often six to 12 months), so feedback is less timely than rate or review indicators.

Dealing with physician reluctance to give up chart review

The biggest obstacle to successfully using review, rate, and rule indicators is physician reluctance to really let go of chart review. Although a peer review committee may label an indicator as a rule or a rate, it may still end up reviewing and discussing every case before sending the automatic rule letter or aggregating the data into a rate. Unfortunately, this reflects a fundamental misunderstanding about what it means to designate a performance measure as a review, rule, or rate indicator. The designation of an indicator as review, rule, or rate establishes up front whether physician chart review will be the first step in evaluating physician performance for that measure.

The Joint Commission standards are driving the need to use more aggregate data to measure physician performance. Using physician chart review for the majority of your physician performance measurements where rule and rate indicators are more appropriate is not only inefficient and unfair, but it also won't get you the data you need for effective compliance.

Understanding and Improving Risk-Adjusted Data

When physicians are given feedback data about outcomes, a common response is, "My outcomes are worse because my patients are sicker." This concern is legitimate and should be addressed by using data adjusted for the severity of the patients' illnesses or other risk factors, such as smoking or obesity. Because of the increasing public availability of hospital-level risk-adjusted data, it is even more important that medical staffs use it at the physician-level whenever possible to improve both the data and physician performance.

Risk-adjusted data compares the actual outcomes to the expected outcomes based on the risk factors available and the pool of patients in the database. The results may be expressed either as the difference (or variance) between the actual and expected outcomes or as the ratio between the actual outcomes divided by the expected outcomes. In the latter method, 1.0 represents the situation where the actual outcomes are the same as the expected outcomes, any number greater than 1 (e.g., 1.1) represents worse than expected, and any number less than 1 (e.g., 0.9) represents better than expected.

There are two main ways to account for risk factors. The first is to use electronic patient information data sets that have already been collected for other purposes. For example, CMS and several proprietary vendors provide risk-adjusted mortality data based on Medicare and state billing databases. These databases use statistical methods to adjust the outcomes for factors that were captured electronically, such as age, diagnoses, procedure codes, and admission sources. Although easy to obtain and less expensive, this information is limited to the factors that were captured electronically and often does not include relevant clinical information.

The other way is to decide which clinical factors (e.g., blood pressure, prior episodes of heart failure) might predict outcomes based on clinical studies or expert opinion. This information is then entered manually into an electronic database and submitted to a central database for statistical risk adjustment. The Society of Thoracic Surgeons' database for cardiovascular surgery is an example of this approach. This method produces more accurate adjustments and better physician attribution but is more labor-intensive. However, with the increasing implementation of electronic medical records, this data may be more easily obtained in the future.

Regardless of what method is used to make risk adjustments, remember that if physicians don't document the existence of a particular risk factor, there is no way to adjust for it. There are a number of approaches to prompt physicians to document patient diagnostic information in ways that can be accepted by the coding staff. The coding professionals have specific external requirements that only allow them to code a disease or complication if the correct words are used by the physician as part of the written medical record. While it is sometimes a source of frustration to physicians that the coders seem to be speaking a different language, by cooperating with the coders through a few simple adjustments, physicians can account for how sick their patients really are.

Using Perception Data to Evaluate Physician Performance

As medical staffs have moved toward implementing measures of all six core competencies, they have found that not all of the data can be obtained from the medical record. As a result, the need to use perception data has increased.

Perception data differs from clinical data in that it is based on how others view your performance in areas that are relatively subjective, such as communication. Although you might think that you are communicating clearly to someone, it is really that person's perception of the clarity of the message that counts. For example, a physician might discuss potential complications of a procedure in precise technical language with a patient who doesn't understand what the physician is saying but doesn't feel comfortable asking questions. The physician leaves the room feeling the conversation has gone well. The patient, however, may have a different view.

Perception data is not entirely new to physician performance measurement. Incident reports and complaints are essentially single-event perception data. As physicians, we may be used to getting some feedback from our physician peers, although some members of a medical staff may object to anyone telling them anything about their practice and their behavior. The big shift in perception data collection that residency programs made was soliciting information from nonphysician clinical staff members.

There are two main types of perception data: passive and active. Passive perception data is data that was not specifically solicited. Examples of passive data are incident reports, complaints, and compliments. This data is typically based on individual events. Active perception data is obtained by the user of the data by soliciting the information from an individual or a group. Examples of active data are evaluation forms, focus groups, survey forms, and survey interviews.

Active methods for collecting perception data have several advantages over passive methods because specific questions can be asked to evaluate specific expectations, data can be aggregated from many individuals to minimize the potential for personal bias of a single individual, and data can be compared to the norm of a group to decrease interpretation bias.

Many physicians already may receive aggregate perception data from patient satisfaction data collected by their medical group or hospital. However, the broader use of these data for evaluating competency will create some discomfort, if not outright pain, for many physicians who are not used to including the opinions of nonphysicians in their performance evaluation. Another frequent concern is whether the survey perceptions are being attributed to the correct physician. We will discuss this further in Chapter 8.

An organization may also use perception data when objective data are not available or are difficult to collect. For example, an organization could measure physician responsiveness to nursing calls by having nurses keep a log of every call time and response time, or the medical staff could send out a survey asking nurses how they perceive the responsiveness of individual physicians. Although the first method is more objective and appears more accurate, getting nurses to remember to record all the call times is often difficult and, ultimately, the organization may obtain little or no data. The perception survey, although not objective, would probably still identify the physicians who are less responsive with much less effort. Figure 5.3 is an example of a perception survey for residents—sent to the clinical staff—regarding physician communication and professionalism that could easily be adapted for attending physicians.

One question often asked is whether peer review of individual cases is considered perception data. Although peer review may appear to be a subjective process—and, therefore, classified as perception data—in actuality, it is not. Because case review is retrospective, the peer review committee does not actually observe the actions or behavior of the physician under review. Whether the peer reviewer bases his or her decision regarding the care on objective clinical standards or by a consensus of subjective standards, he or she conducts the evaluation using secondary information.

MEASURING PHYSICIAN PERFORMANCE: WHAT TO MEASURE AND HOW TO DO IT FAIRLY

5.3 Sample Resident Survey Tool

Professionalism Assessment Tool

1	2	3	4	5
poor	fair	good	very good	excellent

Please use this scale to rate professionalism during the most recent experience with your resident physician. Circle your answer for each item below.

The physician:

1.	Is approachable	1	2	3	4	5
2.	Takes a genuine interest in the patient's health	1	2	3	4	5
3.	Explores patient's needs and concerns	1	2	3	4	5
4.	Listens carefully	1	2	3	4	5
5.	Answers questions from patients and families	1	2	3	4	5
6.	Communicates clearly and effectively	1	2	3	4	5
7.	Maintains patient's privacy during exams	1	2	3	4	5
8.	Shows compassion and care	1	2	3	4	5
9.	Shows respect for patients and families	1	2	3	4	5
10.	Involves patient/family in decision-making process	1	2	3	4	5
11.	Maintains appropriate behavior with patients and families	1	2	3	4	5
12.	Has good hygiene (e.g., washes hands, wears clean clothes)	1	2	3	4	5

CHAPTER 5

Case Study: Selecting the Right Indicator

Clinical scenario: An 18-year-old primigravida female presents in active labor at full term. She has been followed by her nurse-midwife and has had an uneventful prenatal course. She does well until the second stage of labor, when the nurse-midwife notes a lack of beat-to-beat variability on the fetal monitoring strip and occasional periods of fetal bradycardia. The OB-GYN attending is consulted and decides to use the vacuum extractor and cut a medio-lateral episiotomy to deliver the baby expeditiously. A 6-lb. girl is delivered with meconium aspiration that is successfully treated with oxygenation and vigorous suction. The mother is fine except for a fourth-degree vaginal tear that requires four-layer repair and closure. Mother and baby are discharged after two days of observation. The mother does not experience any urinary or fecal incontinence but does experience a moderate amount of pain from her vaginal tear, as well as pain during intercourse for several months.

Review indicator: Unexpected complication (4th degree laceration)

Questions to reviewer: Could the laceration have been avoided? Was the repair appropriate?

Initial reviewer rating: Care appropriate

Basis for rating: The physician demonstrated timely and appropriate clinical decision-making under difficult circumstances.

Peer review committee discussion: The committee agrees with the initial reviewer findings and commends the OB-GYN attending for delivering a baby in obvious fetal distress so expeditiously. The committee says the inadvertent complication did have an effect on the patient (dyspareunia and generalized pain) but the overall care was appropriate.

The committee also discusses the indicator that triggered the review and notes that third- and fourth-degree lacerations can happen with the best of clinicians and the issue is related to the frequency of episiotomies. The committee recommends to the obstetrics department that it use a rate indicator for third- and fourth-degree lacerations and consider developing a rule indicator for non-indicated episiotomies based on American College of Obstetricians and Gynecologists' (ACOG) data.

Lessons learned: Utilizing a generic indicator such as "unexpected complication" opens a plethora of opportunities for case review, most of which will not yield significant opportunities for improvement.

Refining indicators to specific higher-risk issues or aggregating data into frequency indicators (rates) or quantitative indicators (rules) will significantly decrease a peer review committee's workload.

Monitoring an outcome measurement such as a fourth-degree tear may not have as strong an impact as addressing the process underlying that rate, in this case non-indicated episiotomies. The issue is not whether fourth-degree vaginal tears occur as a result of episiotomies (we know they do approximately 0.6%–4% of the time, depending on the use of forceps or suction and the position of the mother), but whether the obstetrics department wants to reduce the number of non-indicated episiotomies over time. This quality indicator should ideally be driven by the obstetrics department based on the ACOG 2006 guidelines and standards, and not by management or the peer review committee itself.

REFERENCE

1. Donabedian, A. *Evaluating the quality of medical care*, Milbank Memorial Fund Quarterly 44, no. 3 (Jul. 1996 Suppl.): 166–206.

Case Review: Reducing Bias and Improving Reviewer Efficiency and Effectiveness

Although the peer review process is more than just case review, case review is still the foundation of much of peer review. Medical staffs have been doing case review for a long time; however, this doesn't mean they have always done it well. In the course of my consulting work, I find tremendous variation in the effectiveness of case review among medical staffs—even within the same medical staff. Many times, the root of the problem is the medical staff's reluctance to establish a well-defined process built on sound principles to reduce bias. Instead, they often will adhere to tradition (i.e., "We've always done it this way"), even if that way is flawed.

A good case review system should have three main goals:

- Efficiency: Don't waste physician time

- Effectiveness: Find meaningful improvement opportunities

- Fairness: Minimize process biases

This chapter will describe how you can achieve these goals.

Standardizing the Case Review Process

While some of the improvements to the peer review process are based on moving to a multi-specialty peer review structure, as discussed in Chapter 4, no matter which peer review structure you use, the fundamental steps for the case review process remain essentially the same:

- Case identification and screening

- Physician reviewer assignment

- Physician review and initial case rating

- Initial committee review and physician input

- Committee decision and improvement opportunity identification

- Communication of findings and follow-up accountability

Each of the steps presents an opportunity for bias to enter into the process and an opportunity for the medical staff to minimize it. The flow diagram in Figure 6.1 illustrates a typical case review process that tries to minimize bias.

Case Identification and Screening

The first step is to identify cases that qualify for physician chart review. Cases are generally identified in two ways: Screening work lists and referrals. Screening work lists are generated from information systems queries looking for an outcome (e.g., mortality, complications, and readmissions) that can be identified by medical records abstracting and coding. These cases are then reviewed by the peer review staff to determine whether the outcome was potentially related to physician care. This method can be productive if the data identifying the event has a reasonably specific serious outcome (e.g., mortality). When the event is identified by less-specific identifiers (e.g., general complication codes) then these work lists can be quite time-consuming and may not yield useful review cases.

The second method of case identification is through referrals. Here cases are identified as a result of the hospital's various occurrence reporting systems, including patient complaints and risk management incident reports from nursing, hospital departments, case managers, and other physicians. This is more efficient than screening work lists to identify cases but relies on a strong reporting or referral culture to make it work.

Whether cases are identified through work lists or referrals, one of the best ways to reduce bias in case identification is through the development of clear case review criteria. Unless the medical staff defines specific criteria for case review, case referrals become subjective (e.g., "I am concerned about this case"). This leads to the perception, and often the reality, that the cases selected for peer review are biased against the physicians that the medical staff doesn't like. A good case review criterion goes beyond the general issue (e.g., unexpected death). It also defines not only what clinical situations should be included for physician review because of a likelihood that a physician care issue may have contributed to the outcome, but also what clinical situations do not need physician review because it is obvious the review would say the care is appropriate (e.g., death of a patient admitted for palliative care). Often these criteria are in the head of an experienced peer review coordinator. Getting them down on paper for medical staff approval and improvement will reduce the perception of bias and increase inter-rater reliability. Figure 6.2 provides a sample list of review criteria.

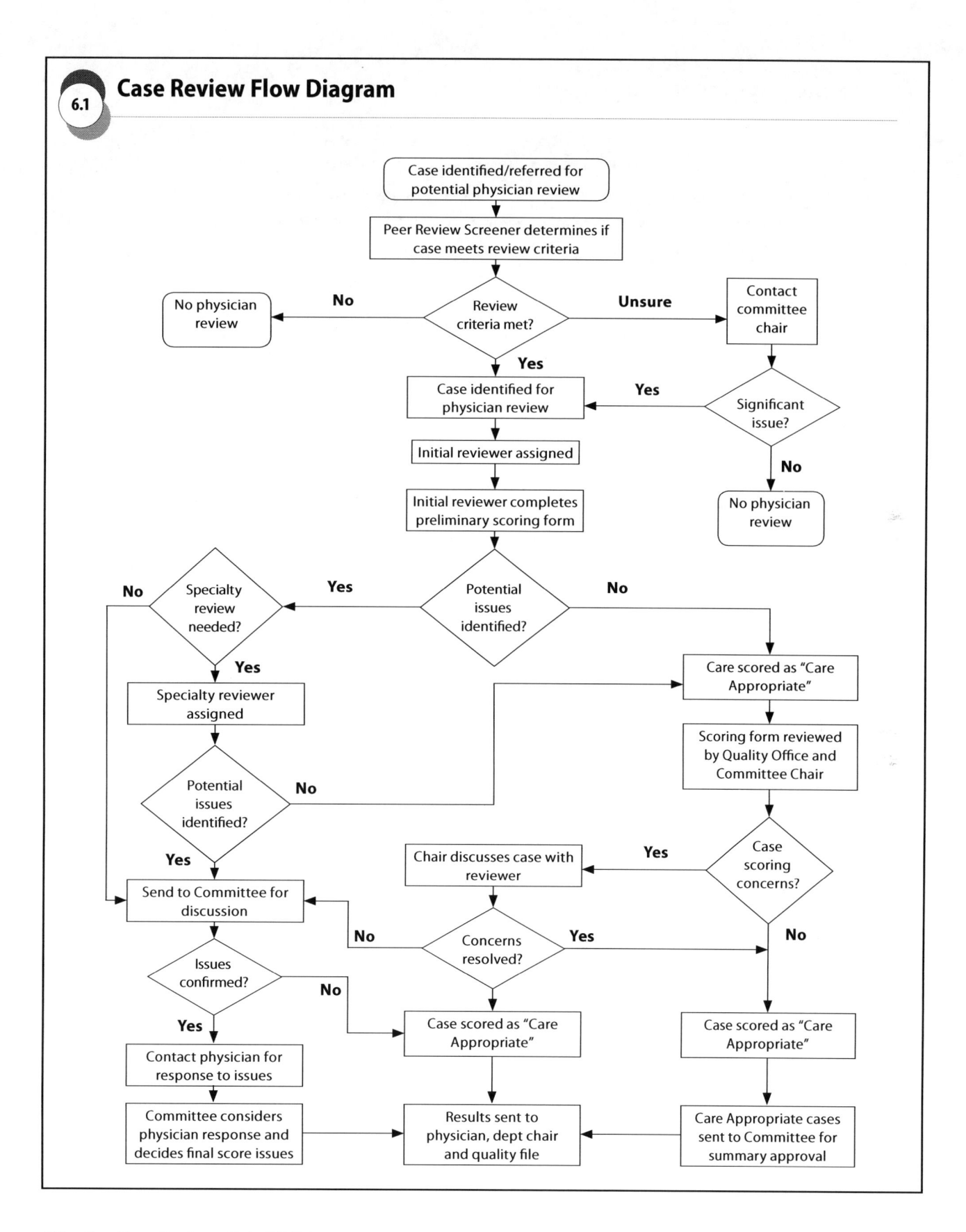

CASE REVIEW: REDUCING BIAS AND IMPROVING REVIEWER EFFICIENCY AND EFFECTIVENESS

6.1 Case Review Flow Diagram

6.2 Improving Case Review Criteria

This table provides examples of how common generic review indicators can be refined by the medical staff through explicit inclusions and exclusions to ensure consistency and fairness in the case screening process and reduce the number of unnecessary reviews. This list is meant to be illustrative and does not represent a complete set of review indicators. Also, each medical staff needs to decide whether the inclusions or exclusions are acceptable for its peer review program.

Indicator	Inclusions	Exclusions
Unanticipated death: Surgical/procedural	Periprocedural mortality or death within 30 days of initial procedure	Procedures for palliative care; patients with unsalvageable clinical findings; procedures with known expected death rates (e.g., cardiac surgery)
Unanticipated death: Medical	Death of inpatient admitted for treatment of medical conditions	Inpatient admissions for palliative care; ED deaths of patients presenting in cardiorespiratory arrest; medical conditions with known expected death rates (e.g., CHF, acute AMI, pneumonia)
Unanticipated death: OB/neonatal	Maternal death, newborn or intrapartum fetal death with gestational age greater than 28 weeks	Infants with severe congenital anomalies
Major complications of inpatients undergoing surgical procedures	Perioperative/post complications occurring either during initial stay or requiring readmission: perioperative cardiac arrest, acute MI, central neurological deficit, respiratory/renal failure, PE, severe sepsis; unplanned removal of an organ; return to OR for evisceration, organ repair, or removal of foreign body	New acute MI during cardiology rescue procedures; return to OR for failed dialysis access, unrelated procedures, planned returns, or a specific complication monitored by rule and rate indicators (e.g., bleeding or hematoma)

6.2 Improving Case Review Criteria (cont.)

Indicator	Inclusions	Exclusions
Major complications of inpatients admitted for medical conditions	Complications occurring either during initial stay or requiring readmission: DVT; PE; medication prescribing errors; unanticipated bleeding; sepsis unrelated to primary diagnosis; neurovascular deficit not present on admission	Routine complications from medications not requiring significant change in treatment plan; adverse drug reactions not due to prescribing errors; adverse reactions to blood product; patients placed on appropriate prevention and therapeutic protocols (e.g., stroke, DVT)
Major maternal peripartum complications	Post-delivery maternal readmission within 7 days; eclampsia; mother transferred to ICU post-delivery; maternal intra- or peripartum blood loss (transfusion of >3 units); post-delivery hysterectomy	Transfusion for abruptio placenta or placenta previa; mothers in ICU pre-delivery; complications monitored by rates (e.g., third/fourth degree lacerations)

These criteria have two uses. The first is to determine which cases need to reviewed by a physician. This is called case screening. Once your organization identifies the cases and has them in hand, typically in the quality department, they are prescreened by quality analysts who often have nursing backgrounds. Because case review indicators are triggered by complex events, this review helps ensure that the issues are potentially physician-related. The quality staff should complete this screening process within a week of its receipt of the chart.

The second use is to improve referrals. Once you have criteria set, don't keep them to yourself. Disseminating the criteria to the likely referral sources will improve the number and quality of the referrals. The most common reason for a low number of case referrals for peer review is that the referral sources don't know what you are looking for. Ideally, referral criteria should be embedded in information systems used by the referral sources (e.g., case management systems or risk management reporting). But criteria also can be available in risk management report forms or on paper in the form of lists for nurse managers or health information management coders.

CHAPTER 6

Physician Reviewer Assignment

Once a case is determined to require physician review, in essence, this is when "peer review" actually begins. For purposes of this book, we will use the term "screener" for what the quality staff does and "reviewer" for what the physician does. At this point two questions need to be addressed:

1. Which physician(s) should be assigned to the review?

2. What do they need to know?

Cases can be assigned for initial review in several ways. They can be automatically assigned to committee members on a rotating basis, by specialty, or by the committee chair after he or she conducts an initial assignment. In the multi-specialty committee model, the rotating assignment or "batting order" approach is often used to reduce specialty bias. Rather than determining the physician reviewer on a case-by-case basis, a predetermined batting order reduces the perception of personal bias in case assignment and also enhances reviewer anonymity because the physician under review can't assume a particular member of the committee was the reviewer.

Of course, if the case has clear technical issues that the next person up in the order can't address, define a method for choosing a pinch hitter in your peer review policy. For example, if the concern in an obstetrics case was whether the fetal monitoring strip was read correctly, clearly that case needs to be assigned to an obstetrician for review.

The one method I do not recommend, regardless of the committee model, is having all case assignments determined by an individual, either the quality staff or the committee chair, on a case-by-case basis. This approach can lead to the perception of personal bias in case assignment.

Another factor that affects case assignment is reviewer conflict of interest. This topic was discussed earlier in Chapter 1. Through either recognition by the case screeners or disclosure by the assigned reviewer, case assignments must be modified when an automatic or substantial potential conflict is identified.

Once you have determined who should review the case, the next question is with what information should the reviewer be provided. To not waste valuable physician reviewer time, reviewers need to have four pieces of information:

CASE REVIEW: REDUCING BIAS AND IMPROVING REVIEWER EFFICIENCY AND EFFECTIVENESS

1. Why was the case selected for review? This means providing the reviewer with the review criteria, such as unexpected death.

2. What is the clinical scenario? Here the peer review coordinator provides a brief paragraph regarding the key clinical milestones in the case.

3. Which physicians are under review? The peer review coordinator should provide the reviewer with his or her best understanding of which physician's care is raising a concern. However, this should not restrict the reviewer from evaluating other physicians' care if the review leads to it.

4. What questions or concerns need to be addressed? The peer review coordinator should prompt the physician reviewer to address key issues the coordinator has identified. This helps reduce the professional bias of the physician reviewer. Obviously, the reviewer might identify other issues, but he or she must at least address the quality staff's concerns.

Once you identify a case for physician review, you need to have a timely system for putting it in the hands of the reviewer and obtaining an initial assessment. Regardless of how you assign cases, you must do so quickly, ideally within a week after the quality department has received the chart. Similarly, there needs to be a clear time frame for the initial physician reviewer to review the case. Typically, the reviewer should complete his or her review within two weeks of receiving the chart, and at least three days before the peer review committee meeting, to give the meeting members time to prepare.

Physician Review and Initial Case Rating

The physician reviewer's job is to either determine the care is appropriate or provide the basis for a productive discussion at the committee meeting. This is accomplished by actual review of the medical record. This may seem obvious but I have seen peer review programs where the physician merely reviews a detailed summary prepared by the quality staff and the discharge summary by the physician.

While physicians are used to looking at medical records, they often have not received any clear instruction on what they should be looking for when performing peer review. Figure 6.3 provides some guidance on how this should be done.

6.3 Sample Questions for Chart Reviewer to Use

The primary question a physician reviewer is trying to answer is whether a physician's actions and decisions were appropriate independent of the outcome of care. The two components of this process are identifying the key issues of the case and understanding the provider's rationale. Described below are some questions for the reviewer to consider that will help with each of these tasks.

Guide to physician-care issue identification:

- Was an important diagnosis not considered?

- Was an important procedure, medical treatment, or test not indicated or inappropriate at the time performed?

- Was an important procedure, medical treatment, consultation, or diagnostic test not performed that should have been?

- Was there a problem with procedural technique?

- Was there a delay in diagnosis, evaluation, consultation, intervention, or decision-making that affected the patient's clinical condition?

- Was there a problem with communication, coordination of care, or supervision that affected the patient's clinical condition?

Guide to understanding the physician's rationale:

- Was the documentation sufficient to understand the rationale for the actions or decisions?

- Did the rationale make good clinical sense at the time?

- Was it consistent with evidence-based medicine or good practice?

- Was it consistent with medical staff expectations? If there is no clear expectation, does the medical staff need to create one?

- Are there technical issues beyond your expertise?

CASE REVIEW: REDUCING BIAS AND IMPROVING REVIEWER EFFICIENCY AND EFFECTIVENESS

Once the record has been reviewed, the reviewer's job has three components:

1. Make an initial judgment of the appropriateness of the overall care and any specific care issues

2. Provide a justification for that opinion (whether or not the care is appropriate)

3. Determine what questions to ask the physician under review that would help fully understand the provider's actions and rationale

Requiring the reviewer to justify his or her opinion and define the initial questions for the provider under review allows for efficient and thoughtful discussion at the committee meeting and makes it less likely that decisions will be made without sound information. Requiring content-based opinions is a good means of reducing the potential for personal bias.

What if an initial reviewer is uncertain regarding the case? If the reviewer understands the issues but is uncertain about whether the care is appropriate, the case should be sent to committee for discussion. However, if the reviewer lacks the expertise to perform the review completely, your organization should make every effort to obtain the appropriate expertise, if possible, before the committee meets. Figure 6.1 illustrates this process.

Initial reviews should always be completed before they go to the committee, typically a few days ahead of time. The first time the initial reviewer looks at a case should not be at the meeting. Although you might hesitate to set a specific time frame for physicians who are volunteering their time, I have found that once the expectation is set by the medical staff and reinforced by the committee chair, most physicians will perform the reviews in advance and in a timely manner. This standard prevents wasting the committee's time and is fairer to the physician under review.

A key factor in achieving good reviewer inter-rater reliability is to use a good case scoring system. This will be discussed later in this chapter along with case studies on case review, which will illustrate how to apply a case scoring system.

As was discussed in Chapter 2, the reviewer should also be looking for exemplary practices as part of the peer review process. In addition, often times there are systems issues that are the root cause of the patient's outcome or have contributed to the decisions made by the physician. These should also be addressed by the reviewer and presented to the committee for discussion.

CHAPTER 6

Initial Committee Review and Physician Input

If the initial reviewer's rating is "care appropriate," then these cases should only be reported to the peer review committee for summary approval. This will focus the committee's time on the important cases.

The concern that is sometimes raised by this approach is the potential for underscoring by the initial reviewer. Medical staffs often worry that cases will be incorrectly rated "care appropriate" and will slip through the cracks, perhaps due to inexperienced or biased reviewers. To address this, I recommend using the committee chair as a secondary reviewer by having him or her review the completed case review form (not the chart) and discuss the case with quality staff members a few days prior to the committee meeting to ensure that the review addressed the key issues and the rationale was sound. If there is a concern, the chair can discuss it with the reviewer and decide whether the case should still be presented. Figure 6.1 illustrates this approach.

If the initial physician reviewer thinks the care was less than appropriate, the case should be placed on the agenda for discussion at the next committee meeting. At this point, the committee should come to one of three conclusions:

1. Confirm the reviewer's concerns and finalize the questions for the provider.

2. Determine additional technical expertise is needed and obtain it prior to the next meeting.

3. Decide that the concerns were not warranted and the care was appropriate. If the latter is the case, the committee might also briefly discuss how that decision might apply to future cases or create a new exclusion criterion if warranted.

After the initial case presentation and before the discussion begins, it is critical to identify and manage potential conflicts of interest. Having the chair ask committee members about any additional disclosures reduces potential perceptions that the committee is biased.

To prevent the potential for bias in the case determination, unless the care is determined to be appropriate, the committee must always ask the physician under review for his or her input prior to making a final determination. Even if the answer seems obvious, peer review requires a due process to be fair. Rushing to judgment prior to requesting input—even if it is clinically correct—can lead to a punitive perception of the committee. One way to avoid that trap is restricting the initial discussion to formulating questions for the provider. This will help the committee stay more open-minded to the requested input.

CASE REVIEW: REDUCING BIAS AND IMPROVING REVIEWER EFFICIENCY AND EFFECTIVENESS

If the committee thinks the care might have been something other than appropriate, it must communicate its concerns to the physician. This is typically accomplished through a letter of inquiry that must inform the physician of the key questions and request a response within a specific time frame (usually two to three weeks). The letter should indicate that failure to respond will result in the committee finalizing the rating based on available information without the physician's input. A sample inquiry letter is provided in Figure 6.4.

How the committee asks the questions to the physician under review makes a great deal of difference regarding your peer review culture. Formatting your concerns in a collegial manner will often produce a better response. Don't ask "Why didn't you do X?" Instead, try asking "Did you consider X, and, if so, why did you choose not do this?" This approach is illustrated in the case studies.

Some additional ways to reduce bias at this stage of the process include:

- Protect reviewer anonymity. Whether you contact the provider before or after the committee meets, it is critical that the contact not come from the reviewer. This is to preserve reviewer anonymity. The communication should come from the committee, not from the reviewer, via either the committee chair or the quality staff. Exceptions to this may be in the academic setting or in practice groups in which there is an economic relationship among all the physicians.

- Preserve provider anonymity. At least in the initial discussion and, if possible, throughout the case review process the provider's identity should not be revealed. While the reviewer will obviously know the provider, redacting names from the review form and other documents can increase the perception that the committee is trying to be as objective as possible.

- Minimize personal appearances. Some committees only allow written responses to make the most efficient use of committee time and to prevent the physician from feeling that he or she is being hauled in front of a tribunal.

- Restrict appearances to responses to questions. If the physician does appear, he or she should be asked to respond to the questions received in advance and any others that arise and should not be present for any discussions or deliberations. Remember, this is not a fair hearing panel.

- Maintain the same process for members. Whichever approach your committee uses, be sure it applies the process in the same way for committee members whose cases are reviewed.

6.4 Sample Case Review Inquiry Letter

Dear Dr. _____

The peer review committee of the medical staff reviewed the following case in which you were the attending/consulting physician.

Patient name:

Chart #:

Admission date:

Criteria for review:

Clinical summary:

Based on the information available in the patient's medical record, the preliminary review of the case has raised the following questions that we would appreciate if you could clarify:

-

-

-

We recognize the medical record often does not contain all the information needed to evaluate care in a complex case. Prior to the committee making a determination on the case, we would like to have your input in writing to the above questions to more fully understand the care provided to this patient.

It is the policy of the medical staff that this response is needed within 14 days of the receipt of this letter so the committee can review cases in a timely fashion. If your response is not received in the appropriate time frame, unfortunately, by policy, the committee will have to complete its evaluation without your valuable input. If you have some mitigating circumstance that would preclude you from meeting this time frame, please contact the quality management department immediately.

Sincerely,

Peer review committee

CASE REVIEW: REDUCING BIAS AND IMPROVING REVIEWER EFFICIENCY AND EFFECTIVENESS

Committee Decision and Improvement Opportunity Identification

After receiving the physician's response, or after the deadline has passed, the committee now can discuss the case and finalize the case rating. Oftentimes, the members may not remember the keys issues of a case from month to month. Since members need to vote, they should have all available information at hand. This means providing every member with copies of the initial review forms, the letter of inquiry, and the provider's response at the meeting. This information is often also made available for viewing in the medical staff or quality office in advance of the meeting.

Remember to take a formal vote on the rating of each case. This is a decision that will be going into a physician's quality file and it requires that level of formality. Also, if the rating system has other elements in it, such as physician care issues or physician contribution to patient harm, remember to have the committee finalize those as well at this time.

It is important to rate each case independent of past cases. Committees should be like an umpire, calling each pitch without regard to the ball and strike count. After the case rating is determined, then it is appropriate to consider whether issues have occurred and the provider's identity can be revealed.

Determining "how many is too many" should not be arbitrary. Set a predetermined number of cases or targets for each level in your rating system that would require a focused review. We will discuss targets further in Chapter 9. Exceptions for focused review should always be made for a single, egregious case.

Unfortunately, most peer review committees stop at this point. However, to move toward an improvement-focused peer review culture, it is important that the committee goes beyond just rating the care to identifying what could be done better in the future; otherwise the committee may be viewed as simply labeling care rather than improving it. Since it came to a conclusion that the care was less than appropriate, the committee has to discuss what should be done differently to prevent similar events and why. The process of transmitting this information to the physician provides the basis for physician self-improvement, which is a primary goal of peer review. The case studies at the end of this chapter illustrate how the committee can perform this function well. However, please note that this is not the same as taking more intentional action, which will be discussed in the next section.

The peer review committee should also identify opportunities for improvement from a systems perspective. Often a case will initially seem to highlight a deficiency in individual physician performance but, upon examination, it turns out to be a problem in another area of care providers, such as nursing or pharmacy. These issues should be brought to the committee for discussion to confirm the need for system improvement.

Communication of Findings and Follow-Up Accountability

The committee should notify the physician whose case is being reviewed of the finding even if the care was appropriate. Communicating all outcomes of the review process to the physician—not just the bad ones—gives the physician a more balanced perspective of the committee's findings. Only contacting physicians when there is bad news leaves the impression that the committee is interested only in the bad apples. Of course, this applies only to cases that have undergone physician review. If a case that does not meet screening criteria is eliminated by the quality staff, there is no need to inform the physician since it never was under peer review.

When care is found to be less than appropriate, the committee must determine the next step to improve the physician's performance. This could range from sending an educational letter regarding the issues and recommended best practices to developing an informal or formal plan. This is where the responsibility typically shifts from the committee to the department chair. The committee informs the department chair of the findings, improvement opportunity, and the need for something more than just a letter. This can range from an informal conversation with the physician to ensure he or she understands the nature of the improvement and agrees to pursue it or to more formal improvement plans and monitoring, which will discussed in Chapter 10.

It is best that improvement plans or other actions are done by a party not involved in the evaluation. This is why department chairs are often not members of peer review committees—to "keep their powder dry." If the chair needs assistance with such a plan, the best candidates to offer it are the vice president for medical affairs, the medical staff officer, or the peer review committee chair.

Many department chairs perform their improvement responsibilities well. Unfortunately, some are allowed to avoid them. If that is the case, your medical staff might perceive the system as unfair. The peer review committee needs a mechanism to ensure that the department chair has created and implemented an improvement plan as well as a policy for what to do if the improvement plan is not met in any way.

CASE REVIEW: REDUCING BIAS AND IMPROVING REVIEWER EFFICIENCY AND EFFECTIVENESS

Case Rating Systems

The main reason for using a scoring system for case reviews is fairness. A scoring system lends itself to more clearly defined thresholds for focused review and allows the medical staff to set prospective targets and address different levels of concerns.

The Greeley Company has consistently advocated for categorical scoring of case reviews. This results in more consistent ratings among reviewers. It also lends itself to database tracking and easier pattern recognition.

This Greeley scoring system is based on the following three principles:

1. Use categories that focus on one aspect of evaluation. Doing so makes scoring easier and more reliable. It is better to have one category that evaluates the potential clinical outcomes and a second category that evaluates the appropriateness of physician care rather than a single category that tries to combine both (e.g., "moderate effect on the patient but no physician care issues"). Likewise, it is important to have a separate category for documentation deficiencies because they are different from technical quality-of-care issues.

2. To rate appropriateness of care, use at least three levels. This allows for the reality of grey areas in case review. With only two levels, even when a physician reviewer disagrees somewhat with the approach taken by the physician under review, the reviewer will tend to score care as "appropriate" if the only other option is "not appropriate."

   Previous editions of this book, recommend the three levels be labeled as: appropriate, questionable (or controversial), and not appropriate. However, I have found that these terms sometimes may contribute to a perception of a punitive culture. As a result, I encourage clients to switch to the terms: no improvement opportunity, minor improvement opportunity, and significant improvement opportunity. Others have chosen: no variance, minor variance, and significant variance. Again, the important thing is to have three levels, regardless of what you call them.

   I am aware that some consulting organizations advocate a "scoreless" system of "no opportunity for improvement" or "referral to department chair." In actuality, this is really a two-level system and does not distinguish between minor and significant improvement opportunities. As a result, on an ongoing professional practice evaluation report a physician with four minor opportunities looks worse than one with three significant opportunities. This is unfair to the first physician. As a result, I still recommend a three-level system.

One question that has been asked is whether exemplary care should be a fourth level. Because the exemplary practices may or may not involve the physician under review or could come from nonphysician caregivers it seems to make more sense to not add it as its own rating level, and instead recognize it with a separate letter of commendation.

3. Define the reasons care might not have been viewed as appropriate. The Greeley Company uses a separate category to identify physician care issues (e.g., skills, knowledge, judgment, communication, and planning). Systematically defining physician care issues at the time each case is decided allows the medical staff to get to the root cause of physician performance concerns and identify patterns for improvement despite differences in the diseases, procedures, or circumstances of the individual case.

A new category to consider for your rating system is physician contribution to patient harm. The harm rating system looks at actual and potential harm separately using a 0–3 scale for each. The sum of the actual and potential harm yields an overall harm score of 0–6.

As I have begun to use this category with medical staffs, the question has been raised whether evaluating harm due to physician care would be of benefit for your peer review committee. On the positive side, it establishes the importance of the case and prioritizes need-for-improvement actions. On the other hand, evaluating harm is a more difficult decision because it implies causality and often takes additional committee time. At this point, it is a judgment call for your peer review program based on how your medical staff would respond.

In addition to the categorical ratings, a good case review system incorporates other important elements of the case review process to prompt the reviewer. This helps to create consistency between reviewers and efficiency of committee evaluation. Some of those elements are:

- Justification for care-appropriate ratings as well as ratings that have concerns

- Key questions for the provider so the committee can focus its discussion on the important issues

CASE REVIEW: REDUCING BIAS AND IMPROVING REVIEWER EFFICIENCY AND EFFECTIVENESS

- Exemplary care nominations for excellent care despite different clinical situations

- System/process or nursing concerns that are identified in the course of the review

Case Review and the Electronic Age

One of the issues frequently mentioned to me by physicians on peer review committees is the shift to reviewing an electronic health record (EHR) rather than the paper record of the past. This is a bit of a paradox since the EHR is supposed to make data access and management more efficient. Although some physicians indicated that they enjoy the flexibility of being able to do reviews from a location of their choice, most commented that conducting peer review is more time-consuming compared to the paper record.

One might think the obvious solution would be to simply print out a paper version of the record for peer review purposes to save physician time. Unfortunately, with the increasing implementation of the true electronic record, the printouts are not designed to replicate the old paper record. As a result, what may have been a 30-page chart on paper now becomes a printout comprised of hundreds of pages that is cumbersome and difficult to review.

Why did this happen? As in any information system, the system design usually is based on a primary objective related to the majority of the transactions within the system; thus, infrequent transactions may suffer. I believe that is the case with peer review. The main focus of the EHR is to get the data in and have remote access to the data in real time. The infrequent need to review the record in its entirety has suffered in the system designs up until this point.

For those engaged in peer review, the question at this point is what can be done about it? Part of the solution is to find physicians who are comfortable with the EHR and may have developed some strategies that they can teach to the other committee members. The second part of the solution is to go back to your vendor or IT administrator to see whether there are ways that their review process might be better conducted within the current design of your system, and then provide training to your committee members.

A second impact of an EHR is its use in the peer review committee meeting. Here, the adage, "Just because you can doesn't mean you should" comes to mind. At a recent peer-review committee meeting that I attended, the peer review staff thought that having this advanced technology would aid

CHAPTER 6

committee discussion for case review. But with the introduction of any new idea, one always has to look at the pros and cons before assuming that change is better.

At issue here are two principles for an effective peer review committee: The preservation of provider anonymity and the efficient use of committee time. So it raises the question of how does being able to project EHR on screen affect these principles.

In the old days, about three or four years ago, when there was only a paper medical record, the peer review coordinator would bring the chart to the committee meeting and if questions arose that required additional clinical information, either the coordinator or the reviewer would look at the chart to find the relevant data. This preserved provider anonymity. When the electronic record is projected on screen, the provider anonymity is lost.

What about committee discussion efficiency? With paper records, while one individual was looking at the chart to get further information, the rest of the committee was free to continue its discussions on other concerns until the information was available. When the committee projects the medical record, I've observed that the entire committee becomes focused on that issue and until the information is found, further discussion seems to cease.

I am very much a proponent of the use of the EHR and peer review. However, you may want to consider having the EHR available on a laptop—instead of projected on a screen—during a committee meeting so that either the peer review coordinator or the reviewer can look at the record to obtain additional information and then relate this information to his or her colleagues.

Case Study: Who Is in Charge?

Clinical scenario: A 72-year-old female with history of heart failure, hypertension, and diabetes who was readmitted on 12/9/09 for exacerbation of her heart failure. Her normal medications were Captopril, Lasix, and KCL. She had not taken her Captopril or Lasix for the five days prior to admission due to financial reasons. She had gained 7 pounds and presented with edema and shortness of breath. On presentation, her pulse was 120, respirations 26, blood pressure 172/92 and weight 206 pounds. There was 4+ pitting edema to mid-shin bilaterally and rales to the mid-lung level bilaterally. The EKG was unremarkable. The internist treated her with diuretics and KCL.

On 12/10, the patient developed substernal chest discomfort while walking. EKG showed anterolateral ST elevation. Her chest discomfort was unrelieved by sublingual nitroglycerin. Her cardiologist was

CASE REVIEW: REDUCING BIAS AND IMPROVING REVIEWER EFFICIENCY AND EFFECTIVENESS

called and she was taken to the cardiac cath lab where a 99% occlusion of the proximal LAD was found and stented. Her heart failure regimen was adjusted by the cardiologist.

On 12/11, the internist saw the patient on early morning rounds, noted that she was improved, and placed her on oral lasix and KCL. Later that morning, the cardiologist rounded on the patient still noting diffuse rales and switched her back from oral to IV diuretics and KCL. At 2 p.m., the potassium value returned as low, at 3.3, and the internist was called with the results. He noted that since the modifications in the patient's orders were made by the cardiologist, he would defer further treatment of the heart failure to the cardiologist. Later that evening the cardiologist was contacted for further orders for the heart failure and potassium supplementation.

Review indicator: Potential delay in treatment

Key questions for physician reviewer: Was there a delay in treatment by the internist's failure to give orders when called? Who was directing the patient's treatment for heart failure?

Initial reviewer rating: Minor improvement opportunity for the internist.

Basis for rating: The main concern was a delay in addressing an abnormal lab value by the internist.

Peer review committee discussion: The committee agrees there appears to be a delay in addressing the low potassium level. The initial discussion focuses on whether the delay caused any patient harm. Although the committeee feels no harm occurred, the potential for harm existed. The discussion proceeds to determine what additional information is needed from the internist. During the discussion, several committee members say the cardiologist could have communicated better with the internist when he decided to change the orders. The question is raised as to what the policy is for this circumstance. As a result, the committee decides to send inquiry letters to both physicians and the medicine department chair as to whether there was a system issue underlying this occurrence and to determine if a policy exists on this issue.

Questions to the physicians:

To the internist: When you received the call regarding the low potassium level, did you consider adjusting the patient's medications at that time and, if so, why did you choose not to? Did you contact the cardiologist to discuss the case or request the nursing staff inform him of the laboratory values? From your perspective, who was directing the care of the patient's heart failure at that time?

To the cardiologist: From your perspective, who was directing the care of the patient's heart failure? Did you discuss the medication changes with the internist? Did anyone contact you about the low potassium level?

To the medicine department chair: Is there a policy regarding who is the "captain of the ship" when a medical subspecialist and internist are involved in treating the same patient?

Physician responses:

From the Internist:

To the peer review committee,

This letter is in response to your questions. First, as to whether I considered addressing the low potassium level, since the cardiologist had changed the orders to oral potassium, I felt that he was managing the patient's heart failure so I deferred to his judgment on how to address the issue. Second, while I mentioned this to the nurse, I did not put a note in the chart to this regard and I did not contact him directly as I assumed he would be by on rounds shortly. In retrospective, I believe it would have been best for me to contact him to straighten this out.

I do believe that the organization would benefit from having a policy on whether specialists should be modifying orders if they are not requested to do so by the internist. I would be willing to serve on any subcommittee that looks into this issue.

Sincerely,

Internist

From the Cardiologist:

To the peer review committee,

This letter is in response to your questions. While on rounds as a follow-up to the patient's stent procedure the day before, I did modify the patient's medications. However, I did not feel that this constituted acceptance of the management of the patients overall heart failure, which I believe resided with the internist. However, I can see how it may have caused some confusion. I did not discuss the medication changes with the internist directly. I was not contacted about the low potassium level until the evening, at which time I modified the orders.

I feel that we as an organization should have a set policy on who is the captain of the ship. It would make it much easier for specialists to know what they should be handling without feeling like they are interfering with the care provided by others.

Thank you for your inquiry on this case. I hope that we can resolve this issue.

CASE REVIEW: REDUCING BIAS AND IMPROVING REVIEWER EFFICIENCY AND EFFECTIVENESS

Sincerely,

Cardiologist

From the medicine department chair:

To the peer review committee,

At this point there is no written policy on this issue. We have allowed physicians to work these issues out individually to maintain our culture of not being intrusive into medical practice. That said, while that approach may have been useful in the past, with the increased complexity of care today, I believe it would a good time to create such a policy.

Sincerely,

Medicine department chair

Committee discussion and final determination: After reviewing the responses, the committee affirms the initial reviewer's rating of minor improvement opportunity for the internist as an issue with clinical judgment and communication, in that the lab value should have either been addressed at that time or a consultation obtained with the cardiologist. The committee also feels the cardiologist had a minor improvement opportunity in regard to communication when making changes to orders by the primary physician. For both physicians, an education letter is deemed sufficient, which contains an appreciation for their acknowledgment that in hindsight they could have approached the situation differently. Finally, the committee refers to the issue of a captain of the ship policy to the MEC.

Lessons learned:

- Just because the delay did not result in patient harm, this does not affect the need to evaluate the care and identify improvement opportunities. While it is easy for committee's to dismiss cases if there is no harm, peer review needs to remain focused on the physician's actions and decisions regardless of the outcome.

- Through the initial committee discussion, based on the broader perspective of the group, the potential issue regarding the cardiologist's contribution to the confusion was also identified. Even though there was no specific policy, the need to improve communication was addressed.

- When physicians respond to the committee with self-acknowledgment of the need for improvement, the committee should thank them for their openness and collegiality.

CHAPTER 6

- When a system's issue—the lack of a clear policy—is identified, the committee needs to refer this issue to the medical staff entity with policy authority, typically the MEC, rather than trying to resolve the issue itself. Despite the agreement of the parties involved in this case that this would be a good idea, because of the prevailing culture, this will be a complex issues to resolve and needs to start at the highest medical staff level.

7. Selecting Physician-Driven Measures for OPPE: Understanding and Applying the Six Core Competencies

To implement ongoing professional practice evaluation (OPPE), the first question your medical staff needs to answer is "How will we define physician competency?" The second is "How will we measure it?"

Even though this chapter appears to focus on The Joint Commission's requirements for OPPE, it is important to note that the measurement of physician competency is essential as a best practice whether you are part of a hospital medical staff, an ambulatory care setting, an employee or contracted physician group, an independent group practice, or a group of physicians linked by a provider contract (e.g., an accountable care organization). As such, the principles and approaches discussed here are applicable to all those situations.

As discussed in Chapter 2, how your peer review culture views physician competence will affect your answer to the measurement question. Measuring physician quality is often viewed as a difficult, if not impossible, task. However, other industries have found ways to measure quality. Let's look at how they have approached quality measurement to see whether there are lessons that can be applied to healthcare.

When consumer rating services look at quality, they do not treat it as a single entity. Rather, they view quality as the sum of a number of parts. For example, when a consumer guide rates the quality of an automobile, it creates an overall quality rating by first determining the key performance areas that define a quality car and then rating each area. Breaking down the vague concept of a "quality" car to comparisons of engine size, acceleration, interior roominess, seat comfort, exterior design, amenities, warranty, and resale value allows a more reliable estimate of quality than just a summary opinion.

Taking this approach, the definition of quality measurement would be as follows:

To measure quality, quality must be defined in a measurable way.

This may sound a bit circular, but defining the measurable dimensions of performance for a product or service creates the ability to measure quality. Applying this concept to physician competency, to measure physician performance adequately, you need a comprehensive physician competency framework. So how do you define and implement this approach?

It begins by defining the aspects or dimensions of physician performance that are important to your medical staff. When asked about performance, physicians tend to mention good procedure outcomes, low mortalities, low infection rates, appropriate medication use, and accurate diagnoses. However, such expectations represent only one aspect of physician performance: technical quality of care. A comprehensive framework goes beyond that to the broader definition of physician performance discussed in Chapter 1.

ACGME, ABMS, and The Joint Commission: Where Did the Core Competencies Come From and How Are They Used?

The most common physician competency framework currently is the six general or core competencies. This framework was developed by the Accreditation Council for Graduate Medical Education (ACGME) and the American Board of Medical Specialties (ABMS) in the late 1990s and adopted by The Joint Commission in 1997 to help drive OPPE. It was created based on a desire to have more defined methods for evaluating resident competency during training that would go beyond merely measuring technical skills. This framework has six categories:

- Patient care

- Medical knowledge

- Practice-based learning and improvement

- Interpersonal and communication skills

- Professionalism

- Systems-based practice

In understanding these six categories, it should be noted that the ACGME, the ABMS, and The Joint Commission have slightly different definitions. These definitions are shown in Figure 7.1. The differences reflect the perspective of each organization: Residency trainees, actively practicing diplomates, and medical staff–attending physicians. For the most part, there is little difference in the definitions that would substantially change what you might measure for these categories, but there are differences in how you would measure it.

7.1 Core Competency Definition Comparison

	The Joint Commission	American Board of Medical Specialties (ABMS)
Patient care (and procedural skills for ABMS)	Practitioners are expected to provide patient care that is compassionate, appropriate, and effective for the promotion of health, prevention of illness, treatment of disease, and at the end of life.	Doctors must be able to provide patient care, including the safe and effective use of procedures, that is compassionate, appropriate and effective for the treatment of health problems and the promotion of health.
Medical knowledge	Practitioners are expected to demonstrate knowledge of established and evolving biomedical, clinical and social sciences, and the application of their knowledge to patient care and the education of others.	Doctors must demonstrate knowledge of established and evolving biomedical, clinical, epidemiological and social-behavioral sciences, as well as the application of this knowledge to patient care.
Interpersonal and communication skills	Practitioners are expected to demonstrate interpersonal and communication skills that enable them to establish and maintain professional relationships with patients, families, and other members of healthcare teams.	Doctors must demonstrate interpersonal and communication skills that result in the effective exchange of information and collaboration with patients, their families, and health professionals.
Professionalism	Practitioners are expected to demonstrate behaviors that reflect a commitment to continuous professional development, ethical practice, an understanding and sensitivity to diversity, and a responsible attitude toward their patients, their profession, and society.	Doctors must demonstrate a commitment to carrying out professional responsibilities and an adherence to ethical principles.
Systems-based practice	Practitioners are expected to demonstrate both an understanding of the contexts and systems in which healthcare is provided, and the ability to apply this knowledge to improve and optimize healthcare.	Doctors must demonstrate an awareness of and responsiveness to the larger context and system of health care, as well as the ability to call effectively on other resources in the system to provide optimal health care.
Practice-based learning and improvement	Practitioners are expected to be able to use scientific evidence and methods to investigate, evaluate, and improve patient care.	Doctors must demonstrate the ability to investigate and evaluate their care of patients, to appraise and assimilate scientific evidence, and to continuously improve patient care based on constant self-evaluation and lifelong learning.

The key difference in how each organization approached these categories is that in 2000, the ACGME also created specific expectations to be measured in each category. Although specific measures were not mandated, these expectations provided more consistency in the approach to measurement among residency programs.

In contrast, the ABMS did little with this framework until it began to actively encourage its member boards to implement Maintenance of Certification (MOC) in 2008. The ABMS did not actually provide a definition for each category until 2010. In addition, rather than creating a standardized set of measurement expectations among its member boards for each category, MOC allowed each board to determine how each category should be measured. Even within a given board, the individual diplomate often has options on which measures to choose to evaluate his or her own competency.

The Joint Commission adopted the six definitions from the ACGME almost verbatim, but it has yet to define the measurable expectations. Instead, it allows the field to determine how to measure each category for OPPE. This has resulted in a great deal of confusion among hospitals regarding what measures apply to each category. For example, some hospitals will place a core measure, like appropriate antibiotic selection for patients with pneumonia, under patient care while others will put it under medical knowledge and others under practice-based learning. The goal of this chapter is to provide a rational approach for choosing measurements through a better understanding of each category and allow medical staffs to consistently apply this framework.

Alternative Frameworks to the Core Competencies

While there are other frameworks that can be used to define physician competency beyond the scope of this chapter (e.g., the Royal College of Physicians and Surgeons of Canada has defined seven physician competencies called CanMEDS©), there is one other well-known framework that should be discussed. This framework was originally taught by the late Howard Kirz, MD, at the American College of Physician Executives courses on managing physician performance in group practices, and later was adopted by The Greeley Company for use by medical staffs. In its current form, it is composed of six physician performance dimensions, defined as follows:

- Technical quality: Skill and judgment related to effectiveness and appropriateness in performing the clinical privileges granted

- Service quality: Ability to meet the customer service needs of patients and other caregivers

- Patient safety/patient rights: Cooperation with patient safety and rights, rules, and procedures

- Resource use: Effective and efficient use of hospital clinical resources

- Relationships: Interpersonal interactions with colleagues, hospital staff, and patients

- Citizenship: Participation and cooperation with medical staff responsibilities

Among the reason medical staffs have chosen this framework are:

- This framework has been used for more than 15 years as a best practice with attending physicians on hospital medical staffs

- The categories may seem more understandable to many attending physicians

- Many medical staffs have already defined expectations for this framework

- By simply creating a crosswalk of how these categories relate to the six core competencies framework, it will meet your accreditation requirement (see Figure 7.2).

7.2 Competency Framework Crosswalk

ACPE/Greeley	The Joint Commission					
	Patient Care	Medical Knowledge	Practice-Based Learning	Interpersonal/ Communication Skills	Professionalism	Systems-Based Practice
Technical Quality	X	X				
Service Quality	X			X	X	X
Patient Safety/ Rights	X			X	X	X
Resource Use						X
Relationships				X	X	
Citizenship			X		X	

CHAPTER 7

Although this book does not advocate conceptually one framework over the other, if you are accredited by The Joint Commission, you must adopt a comprehensive physician competency framework to meet its standards. If you are not Joint Commission–accredited, you still should adopt a physician competency framework because it is a best practice and will provide the basis for rational physician competency measurement.

That said, while other frameworks are useful, because two major physician-led organizations are applying the six core competencies framework to evaluating physician performance and The Joint Commission has adopted it as well, most medical staff are now using this as their physician competency framework. Therefore, the remainder of this chapter will focus on further understanding and applying the six core competencies to improve physician performance.

Using the Competency Statement and Expectations to Drive Physician Performance Measures

Once the framework has been defined, the next challenge is to decide what specific expectations would best help your physicians understand how to achieve excellence in all areas of competency covered by the framework. These expectations then become the basis for selecting performance measures that will provide the data to evaluate the core competencies. The result of this is that, instead of creating a laundry list of indicators, your physician competency measures have a clear context for why you are measuring something and what competency you are trying to improve.

As mentioned above, while the ACGME went through the process of developing expectations for the trainees in their accredited programs, the ABMS and The Joint Commission did not define expectations.

One reason for some of the confusion regarding the six core competencies is that medical staffs sometimes focus only on the category title and ignore or get lost in the category definition. It is helpful to focus on the main issues described in the category definition as a starting point for setting expectations and ultimately for selecting performance measures. Outlined below are the key issues driving each competency category:

- Patient care:
    - Effectiveness
    - Appropriateness

SELECTING PHYSICIAN-DRIVEN MEASURES FOR OPPE

- – Compassion
- Medical/clinical knowledge:
  - – Obtaining the knowledge
  - – Applying the knowledge
- Interpersonal and communication skills:
  - – Written communication
  - – Verbal communication
  - – Cooperation
- Professionalism:
  - – Responsible attitude
  - – Citizenship
- Systems-based practice:
  - – Resource use
  - – Patient safety
- Practice-based learning and improvement:
  - – Improvement
  - – Information technology use

Once you understand the key issues, development of expectations and measures for each category becomes more focused and useful. The next question is "Where do you find these expectations?" Figure 7.3 describes the potential sources of expectations and a practical method to create them. In general, expectation statements should be relatively broad. The specific measures will define the expectation more precisely. The most important thing to remember is that most expectations should be measurable.

7.3 Creating Great Expectations

Step 1: Define physician performance dimensions or general competencies. These include the following:

The Joint Commission/ACGME/ABMS framework

- Patient care
- Medical knowledge
- Practice-based learning and improvement
- Interpersonal and communication skills
- Professionalism
- Systems-based practice

Greeley/ACPE framework

- Technical quality of care
- Quality of service
- Patient safety and patient rights
- Resource use
- Peer and coworker relationships
- Citizenship

Step 2: Select behaviors that define your culture. The following are sources of cultural values and behaviors:

- Bylaws, rules, regulations, policies
- Medical society recommendations
- Leadership experience and vision
- Current common practices
- Other expectations (e.g., ACGME)

7.3 Creating Great Expectations (cont.)

Step 3: Identify key performance issues. Use the following as sources of performance issues:

- Medical staff indicators
- Administrative and staff complaints
- Patient satisfaction data
- Case review findings
- Incident reports
- Leadership experience

Step 4: Articulate each desired cultural and performance behavior as an expectation.

- Have one or two authors prepare a list for discussion
- Perform group triage list for inclusions and exclusions
- Have the author rework controversial expectations
- Discuss revised expectations
- Determine initial list for distribution and feedback

Step 5: Obtain medical staff feedback and approval.

- Obtain medical executive committee (MEC) feedback and modify appropriately
- Distribute to the medical staff for written feedback within a prescribed time frame
- Discuss at either a general medical staff meeting or department meetings
- Modify based on constructive medical staff feedback
- Submit to the MEC for approval

Step 6: Develop a mechanism by which to communicate expectations. This mechanism can include the following:

- Appointment orientation
- Reappointment
- Physician performance feedback

CHAPTER 7

For example, for the patient care competency, one expectation for providing effective care could be as follows:

Achieve patient outcomes that meet or exceed generally acceptable medical staff standards as defined by comparative data, medical literature, or peer review activities.

Figure 7.4 provides examples of medical staff expectation statements for each of the six core competencies.

7.4 Competency Framework

The Joint Commission/ACGME framework

Patient Care: Practitioners are expected to provide patient care that is compassionate, appropriate, and effective for the promotion of health, for the prevention of illness, for the treatment of disease, and at the end of life as evidenced by the following:

- Achieve patient outcomes that meet or exceed generally accepted medical staff standards as defined by comparative data and targets, medical literature, and results of peer review evaluations

- Use sound clinical judgment based on patient information, available scientific evidence, and patient preferences to develop and carry out patient management plans

- Demonstrate caring and respectful behaviors when interacting with patients and their families.

Medical Knowledge: Practitioners are expected to demonstrate knowledge of established and evolving biomedical, clinical, and social sciences, and the application of their knowledge to patient care and the education of others, as evidenced by the following:

- Use evidence-based guidelines when available, as recommended by the appropriate specialty, in selecting the most effective and appropriate approaches to diagnosis and treatment

Practice-Based Learning and Improvement: Practitioners are expected to be able to use scientific evidence and methods to investigate, evaluate, and improve patient care as evidenced by the following:

- Review your individual and specialty data for all general competencies, and use this data for self-improvement to continuously improve patient care

7.4 Competency Framework (cont.)

Interpersonal and Communication Skills: Practitioners are expected to demonstrate interpersonal and communication skills that enable them to establish and maintain professional relationships with patients, families, and other members of healthcare teams as evidenced by the following:

- Communicate clearly with other physicians and caregivers, patients, and patients' families through appropriate oral and written methods to ensure accurate transfer of information

Professionalism: Practitioners are expected to demonstrate behaviors that reflect a commitment to continuous professional development, ethical practice, an understanding and sensitivity to diversity, and a responsible attitude toward their patients, their profession, and society as evidenced by the following:

- Act in a professional, respectful manner at all times to enhance a spirit of cooperation and mutual respect and trust among members of the patient care team

- Respond promptly to requests for patient care needs

- Respect patients' rights by discussing unanticipated adverse outcomes and by not discussing patient care information and issues in public settings

- Participate in emergency room call coverage as determined by medical staff policy

Systems-Based Practice: Practitioners are expected to demonstrate both an understanding of the contexts and systems in which healthcare is provided, and the ability to apply this knowledge to improve and optimize healthcare, as evidenced by the following:

- Strive to provide cost-effective quality patient care by cooperating with efforts to manage the use of valuable patient care resources

- Participate in the hospital's efforts and policies to maintain a patient safety culture, reduce medical errors, meet national patient safety goals, and improve quality

CHAPTER 7

In addition to setting expectations through general statements, the process of setting targets for physician competency measures in itself sets a tangible expectation for physician performance. Chapter 9 will discuss how setting targets can further define expectations and drive a performance improvement–focused peer review culture.

Applying the Core Competencies to OPPE

Once your medical staff or physician group has clarified the expectations of its members, the next step is to implement these expectations in a tangible way. Although not every expectation needs direct measurement, keeping the need for measurement in mind when you are describing your expectations will make them easier to define. Linking physician data to these expectations greatly reinforces the competency framework and the expectations within it.

It is true that expectation statements alone can be a useful tool that excellent physicians will use to guide their approach to patient care without any measurement. For example, some people are good citizens who always follow the posted speed limit. However, for some, if not most individuals, measurement is necessary to ensure and improve performance. For example, although speed limit signs are posted on most roads, we still have police officers who measure performance (and sometimes provide feedback in the form of a speeding ticket). Otherwise, many individuals would likely not comply. In healthcare, when practice guidelines were first measured regarding prescribing ACEI medications at discharge for patients with congestive heart failure, most physicians thought they were in compliance. Then they received their data. Despite good intentions, many physicians were surprised to find they were routinely performing at a lower level than they had assumed.

While it is beyond the scope of this book to classify an exhaustive list of potential physician competency measures by the core competencies, the box on page 117 provides suggestions of how common aspects of physician performance measurement could be classified. Note that it does not define the exact indicator to use, but rather the area of measurement for which one or multiple indicators may be useful. For example, some complications may be measured as rates and others by case review.

Although the list has suggested measures for practiced-based learning, The Joint Commission stopped requiring OPPE measures for this category. This was because hospitals found that, unlike in a residency training setting or a board certification where specific learning can be tracked via testing, those methods were typically not available in a hospital setting. Therefore, while practiced-based learning

GUIDE FOR CLASSIFYING PHYSICIAN PERFORMANCE MEASURES FOR THE SIX CORE COMPETENCIES

Clearly, there can be legitimate debate about which category might best apply to a measure or whether a measure belongs in more than one category. For example, is a physician's availability for emergency department (ED) call an issue of professionalism, as a medical responsibility, or an issue of systems-based practice because it affects the system for providing timely patient care? With that in mind, the goal of this list is to provide some guidance on which measures *seem* to fit the best in each category.

- Patient care
  - Effectiveness
    - Mortality
    - Complications
    - Readmissions
  - Appropriateness
    - Case review ratings
    - Indications for treatments/procedures (medical necessity)

- Medical/clinical knowledge
  - Applying the knowledge
    - Compliance with use of evidence-based medicine
      - Physician-relevant core measures
      - Compliance with medical staff order sets

- Interpersonal and communication skills
  - Written communication
    - Medical record documentation requirements
    - Timeliness of documentation
  - Verbal communication
    - Patient satisfaction/patient complaints

GUIDE FOR CLASSIFYING PHYSICIAN PERFORMANCE MEASURES FOR THE SIX CORE COMPETENCIES (CONT.)

- – Cooperation
    - ○ Non-cooperation with patient care needs

- Professionalism
    - – Responsible attitude
        - ○ Inappropriate behavior
        - ○ Responsiveness
    - – Citizenship
        - ○ Participation in ED call

- Systems-based practice: Potential measures
    - – Resource use
        - ○ Length of stay
        - ○ Cost
    - – Patient safety
        - ○ Compliance with safety policies

- Practice-based learning and improvement
    - – Improvement
        - ○ Improvement on ongoing professional practice evaluation reports
    - – Information technology use
        - ○ Compliance with use of physician electronic health record tools

Physician Data Attribution: Making OPPE Data Meaningful to Individual Physicians

"Begin with the end in mind." This is a well-known quote from the personal improvement guru, the late Stephen Covey. There are two applications of this adage when it comes to physician attribution of performance measures.

The first application is in the design of data systems. When The Joint Commission in the late 1980s began to seek data from hospitals as part of its Agenda for Change, it created software for the hospitals to use in pilot studies to collect the data. Although the indicators were created by task forces largely composed of physicians and often measured aspects of patient care affected by physicians, there was no thought to include the ability to abstract data regarding individual physicians. Similarly, when the Centers for Medicare & Medicaid Services determined hospitals would collect core measure data, there was no requirement for data vendors to provide the ability for the abstracts to attribute care to an individual physician.

The reason for the inadequate capability to create physician-level data in both of these instances was because the organizations driving these initiatives focused on the need for the hospital to improve patient care. What was forgotten was that, if physician practice was a key factor in hospital performance, the hospital would need physician-level data to convince individual physicians that their own practice needed to improve. The consequence of this oversight was that physician-level data often was not available or incorrectly attributed to physicians for several years and physician confidence in their personal data was affected.

The second application of the Covey quote relative to physician attribution is that if your end is that you want physicians to use the data on an individual level, such as in ongoing professional practice evaluations (OPPE), you must begin with engaging physicians in the determination of the correct attribution. This determination must occur before the data is collected. Otherwise, countless hours are wasted trying to get physicians to accept data that does not reflect their individual performance.

CHAPTER 8

The assessment of physicians through OPPE is no different than the assessment of any hospital employee through a personnel evaluation. For example, no quality coordinator wants data in his or her annual evaluation regarding his or her punctuality that is not accurately attributed to the quality coordinator. So why would a physician want his or her competency to be evaluated if the attribution is not reflective of the physician's performance?

The systematic physician engagement in attribution starts at the peer review committee. Just as peer review committees will typically be asked to annually review the indicators used for evaluating physician performance, it is equally important that these committees review and approve the physician attribution assigned to these measures.

As we discuss physician data attribution, we need to keep in mind that patients in hospitals today often present complex cases and are usually cared for by a team of physicians. This makes attribution an even greater challenge than in the past when the primary care physician provided most of the inpatient care. Therefore, there is both art and science involved in this determination. Information system limitations may prevent physicians from getting the optimal attribution precision. The purpose of this chapter is to assist peer review committees and quality staff to work together to make the best possible attribution choices.

To understand this better, we will start by discussing the general approach to using imprecise data. Then we will look at attribution challenges facing case review, process outcome measurement, and patient satisfaction.

Using Imprecise Data for OPPE

Physicians are used to receiving precise data to diagnose and treat their patients. When they send a blood specimen to the clinical laboratory for hemoglobin level to check for anemia, if the value comes back as 7.9 gms/dl, they are pretty confident that the value is 7.9 gms/dl, not 7.8 or 8.0. The sophistication of automated clinical laboratory equipment today provides that degree of precision. But it was not always so when, long ago, before most of us practiced medicine, manual assays were used to measure hemoglobin.

Unfortunately, the precision of data we use today to measure physician performance is more like the manual assays of yesterday than the slick machines of today. Physicians in the past certainly were able to use the data from the manual systems; they just had to be more careful in how they interpreted it.

PHYSICIAN DATA ATTRIBUTION: MAKING OPPE DATA MEANINGFUL TO INDIVIDUAL PHYSICIANS

Similarly, as we begin to work with physician performance data, the first step is to adjust our expectations regarding its precision to obtain the value it can provide. So what should our expectations be today for physician performance data?

First, don't wait for perfect data. The philosopher Voltaire had a quote that I have heard repeated by many surgeons, "Perfect is the enemy of good." In the surgical context, it meant that taking an extraordinary amount of time to do the perfect operation was more risky to the patient than doing a good operation in a much shorter period of time. If we don't act on reasonable outcome data because we are waiting for it to be perfect, we miss the opportunity for improving patient care today rather than several years from now.

This was the case when the Institute of Medicine, in its landmark book in 1999, *To Err is Human,* provided data indicating that between 44,000 to 98,000 patient deaths were due to medical error. Unfortunately, the response of the medical community and organized medicine in particular was to spend its effort questioning the data rather than acknowledging that, whatever the accurate number was, efforts needed to begin immediately to reduce patient deaths.

Moving on to another expectation, you need to address data use up front. When discussing physician attribution, the question often asked is "Can we really use imprecise data?" However, in working with physician measurement over the past 25 years, I have found that physicians are much more concerned about a different question. While physicians pose the question in terms of data precision, the underlying question is really "How will the data be used?" Until the use question is addressed, the precision discussion will be driven by fear and suspicion. This concern is not unique to physicians; it applies to any group whose performance is in part being measured by less-than-precise data.

So how do you address data use? It starts with an acknowledgment that the data is imprecise and any use will require appropriate dialogue and understanding. It continues in how you express the culture values for peer review discussed in Chapter 2. In particular, your approach to understanding the data begins with asking the right question, "Why are you different?" not "Why are you bad?"

Third, look for big differences. This is called the signal-to-noise ratio principle. To illustrate this idea, when I was driving one winter night on the East Coast, I wanted to listen to the Chicago Bulls basketball game, which was on a Clear Channel radio station from Chicago. The radio reception in the car was not perfect, so I assumed I wouldn't be able to get any useful information from it. Yet even with the static, I could easily discern the score of the game and who was making the plays. The signal was stronger than the noise.

Applying this approach to physician performance data, determine whether there is sufficient variance among physicians that it would be reasonable to ask, "Why are some physicians at the bottom while others are at the top?" In other words, before rejecting data as useless because it is imprecise, see whether the data variance provides some signal that needs to be listened to above the noise.

A question related to the signal-to-noise principle that is sometimes raised is "What if the attribution is to the physician but the care is provided by someone under the physician's supervision?" This question is in part due to the lack of nonphysician or trainee attribution choices in the information systems of the past. While this may slowly change with the electronic health record (EHR), there is still some signal in the current data by looking at the variance. What differs is not who the data is attributed to, but how it is interpreted. Rather than assuming the physician's care is inadequate, one would examine whether the supervision provided was appropriate as the underlying cause.

Finally, try to make the data better. This approach recognizes that physician performance measurement is here to stay, so it is in our interest to make it work for us. This is accomplished through two steps. The first is to identify key data error sources. When you are asking the why-are-you-different question, one of the answers will be data error. The next question, then, is, "If this error is happening to this physician, is it also affecting others?" In root cause analysis, this is called transportability. Determining the root cause of data error can lead to better data in the future. Ignoring it will lead to continued frustration and loss of data credibility. The second step is to work to fix data errors. Here the active oversight by the peer review committee can drive this process and require an ongoing dialogue between the sources of data and the users.

Attribution and Case Review

During case reviews, there may be long conversations regarding which physicians contributed to a patient's outcome. From that perspective, certainly attribution is not a trivial issue for case review. However, because the initial physician reviewer and, ultimately, the peer review committee are using the actual medical record to make a determination regarding the attribution of care and obtain physician input to clarify who did what and when, the attribution for case review is quite accurate. For example, when the majority of cases rated minor or significant improvement opportunity appears in an OPPE report, there is rarely any challenge that the cases were attributed to the wrong physician.

Improving Attribution for Process Measures

Process measures, as discussed in Chapter 5, look at whether a specific process occurred, like ordering the correct antibiotic based on national guidelines or whether blood transfusions met pre-determined medical staff criteria. Typically, these processes can be determined by nonphysicians, such as nurses or individuals with some clinical background, and abstracted from the documentation present in the patient's medical record without the need for physician input on a case-by-case basis. The results of process measures may be evaluated by using either a rule or rate indicator approach.

For process measures that are regulatory requirements, like core measures, the abstractors must apply specific rules on what data elements to collect, which patient conditions to include and exclude, and what physician documentation is acceptable. For internal process measures, such as an audit of the use of a specific medication or the timeliness of operative reports, the organization determines how it will collect the data.

The physician attribution challenge for process measures is due to the abstractor's need to enter the data into an information system and that the data is reported to the physician through that system. This leads to the problems described by the two scenarios in the beginning of this chapter. The first issue is the potential for information system limitations facing the abstractor for assigning physician attribution.
The second issue is the lack of oversight by the medical staff of the attribution rules for the abstractors to follow.

Information system limitations initially were due to either the complete absence of attribution fields in the abstracting software programs or inflexibility of the data fields to default values of the attending physician. As hospitals began to recognize the need for physician-level data in the mid-2000s, more organizations demanded that vendors fix these restrictions. Today, most vendor software has the capability to select alternate physician attributions or create a user-defined field to enter them. Unfortunately, I still find some hospital quality staffs that are unaware of these capabilities and believe their attribution choices are
more limited than they actually are. If your quality staff tells your peer review committee that they have information system limitations for physician attribution, ask them to contact their vendor to find out about their real capabilities. If the limitations are real, I suggest you get a different vendor with more up-to-date capabilities.

Today, the greater problem for physician attribution is the lack of medical staff oversight. Take the old Pogo cartoon that intentionally misquoted the famous line of Admiral Perry, "We have met the enemy and he is us." Since abstractors are looking at the actual medical record, for a process measure they have the capability to determine the physician actually responsible for the process. For example, what if the process is an order to be written at the patient's discharge? The abstractor can identify the discharging physician and ascribe it to that physician rather than simply assigning the attribution by default to the attending physician who may not be the one who discharged the patient.

Many quality abstractors, in a desire to be consistent, have developed specific rules for assigning physician attribution. Others, unfortunately, may simply allow the attribution defaults in the software, typically to the attending physician, to define the attribution. Either way, unless the medical staff reviews and approves a set of attribution rules, the accuracy of the attribution can be affected.

Here are some examples of attribution choices for process measures that may vary between medical staffs as well as between the abstractors and the medical staff:

- Aspirin on admission for patients with chest pain: Should the attribution be to the admitting physician, the emergency physician, or the cardiologist? Or does your medical staff have a protocol which allows the emergency department (ED) nurse to give the aspirin without waiting for a physician order?

- ACEI inhibitors prescribed for patients at discharge: Should the attribution be to the attending physician, the discharging physician, or the cardiologist?

- Antibiotics administered within one hour of surgery: Should the attribution be to the surgeon or the anesthesiologist? If the anesthesia provider is a certified registered nurse anesthetist (CRNA), should the attribution be to the supervising anesthesiologist or the CRNA?

- Appropriate antibiotics for community-acquired pneumonia patients: Should the attribution be to the admitting physician, the emergency physician, or the ordering physician (whichever physician that is)?

It may turn out that the quality staff attribution rules were "spot on" in what the medical staff would have wanted. Then the response from the committee would be "Well done, good and faithful servant." But if some of the quality staff's choices do not reflect the view of the medical staff, then the committee's goal is not to beat them up over it, but to use it as an opportunity to move forward with a more accurate set of attribution rules. To engage your medical staff in this critical issue, set a process where your peer review committee annually examines attribution choices for current process measures as well as determines the attribution at the time any new measures are implemented.

An additional factor for process measures that can affect accuracy is physician documentation, either because it is lacking or illegible. Typically, this is due to the inadequacy of documentation, so the abstractors can't determine whether the process met the national guidelines rather than one of attribution. However, physicians often see this as not getting credit for something they did and inaccurately view it as an attribution problem. The true attribution problem related to documentation is legibility. Here the abstractors can't determine the attribution because they can't even read the physician's signature on an order. Hopefully this will be corrected as more organizations implement EHR and computerized physician order entry (CPOE).

What is the future of process measure abstracting and attribution? As hospitals move to an EHR and CPOE, the abstracting for process measures can be potentially automated and achieved by software queries. If this occurs, it is important that the medical staff interacts with the information technology staff to be sure the attribution rules selected for these queries are appropriate.

Outcome Measure Attribution in a Multiple Provider World

Process measures allow a specific action, like a medication order, to be traced to a specific physician. Outcome measures, however, like mortality or complications, can present a greater challenge for accurate physician attribution. As mentioned earlier in this chapter, outcomes may be the result of many processes and often involve multiple physicians, especially with the complexity of patient care in the inpatient setting today. So how can you possibly attribute an outcome measure to a specific physician? Before assuming that the outcome data attribution is inaccurate, it is necessary to ask the following four questions that may make the data more useful.

Has the medical staff been engaged in the definitions of the attribution choices? Most mainframe systems are designed to capture mainly three physician attributions: admitting physician, attending physician, and (less frequently) discharging physician. The admitting and discharging physician are easy to define. However, because the attending physician may change a number of times during hospitalization, this attribution will often be less accurate. Thus, from a data input standpoint, the definitions used for these categories is critical. One reason is the lack of clear definition by the medical staff that will guide the medical record coders on the final determination of the attending. The

second reason is because the care is provided by a group of hospitalists. Here the medical staff needs to consider assigning a group rate to the outcomes data. In that instance, the OPPE reports for each member of the group shows the same data. If the outcome for an aggregate rate reaches the outlier status, the physicians within the group can then determine whether this is due to a specific individual in the group or is based on a specific
clinical practice.

Has the medical staff reviewed and approved the attribution assigned to each outcome measure? While the category attribution definitions will help for data input, there is still the issue of which physician category is chosen for a specific indicator. For example, most outcomes data systems have the option to use the principle surgeon listed in the ICD codes as the physician of interest. Thus, for patients admitted primarily for surgical procedures, it is much better to run the data using this attribution rather than to use the attending physician. Unless the medical staff reviews the attribution being assigned for each indicator, well-intentioned data analysts may choose the wrong attribution.

Is the outcome measure based on an encounter that was predominately with a single physician? Before dismissing outcome data because of general attribution concerns, the medical staff needs to look at the outcome being evaluated to determine whether it is likely to be related to a single physician. For example, outpatient procedures are generally performed by a single physician. Wherever the type of care provided is mainly attributable to a single physician, the medical staff should encourage the data's use in OPPE even if in other settings the same data may not be accurate.

Is there variance in physician results for the specific outcome? As discussed earlier in this chapter, applying the single-to-noise principle for each data is necessary before dismissing the attribution as inaccurate. If there is variance among the physicians being measured, the data should be considered for OPPE if the data evaluation begins with an open mind about the underlying reasons that could be causing the variance.

Attribution and Patient Satisfaction Data

Based on the types of questions typically asked (e.g., How well did my physician communicate to me?), patient satisfaction survey data is a type of process measure. However, it differs from the abstracted process measures previously discussed in that satisfaction data is measuring a perception of the process rather than using clinical data from the medical record. Because the question sums up the perception

PHYSICIAN DATA ATTRIBUTION: MAKING OPPE DATA MEANINGFUL TO INDIVIDUAL PHYSICIANS

of an entire patient encounter rather than a single point in time, the attribution challenges of patient satisfaction data are more like those of outcome data.

As mentioned in Chapter 5, many physicians have concerns about the patient satisfaction data and would like to use the attribution inaccuracy as a basis to dismiss this data out of hand. However, before assuming that all patient satisfaction data attribution is inaccurate, just like with outcome data, it is necessary to ask some questions that might make it useful:

- Was the encounter being measured predominately with a single physician?

- Does the survey identify the physician about whom the patient is being questioned?

- Is there significant variance in physician scores despite the lack of a clear physician designation to the patient?

The first question recognizes that many patient encounters such as ED visits, outpatient procedures, or ambulatory care visits are with a single physician. Since typically the patient is sent a survey regarding that specific encounter, there is little problem with attribution. Similarly, if a patient is admitted for an elective procedure with a relatively short inpatient stay and the surgeon is the only one involved in his or her care, the patient response to the survey will likely be quite accurate.

The second question relates to the survey method. If the survey is done by phone rather than as a mailed written survey, the survey company may be able to prompt the patient about a specific physician who provided most of the care, typically the attending physician or principle surgeon. This can greatly improve attribution. Similarly, for mailed surveys, some vendors are now putting the picture of the main physician on the survey to prompt a more accurate response from the respondent.

The third question requires a more complex analysis of the actual data. As discussed earlier, just because data is imprecise does not mean it is void of useful information. If some physicians are at the top of the curve and others are at the bottom, the attribution may not be precise but there certainly is something worth examining and worth asking the question, "Why are you different?"

Chapter 8

Case Study: Engaging the Medical Staff in Attribution

Scenario: A multi-specialty peer review committee receives complaints from several physicians that the core measure data on their OPPE reports shows a higher volume of patient activity than they expected. The multi-specialty peer review committee requests the hospital quality director to come to its next meeting to discuss how data was being abstracted. The director explains to the committee that the abstractors met last year and discussed how the attribution was to be assigned. For example, aspirin within 24 hours of admission for chest pain was assigned to the admitting physician. However, while the staff had come to a verbal agreement, there was no written description regarding whom to attribute each measure.

The committee requests that a written list of the physician attributions for each core measures be provided for the committee to review at the next meeting. Upon reviewing the list, the committee finds most of the attributions were acceptable but makes changes to several measures on the list. For example, the committee feels that the ED physician is accountable for the aspirin on admission unless the patient is a direct admission and does not go through the ED. The ED director agrees with this approach as well, as he wishes to hold his physicians accountable for this process.

Following the review of the core measures, the committee asks the same process be followed for all rate and rule measures on the OPPE reports. At the next peer review committee meeting, the staff provides a list of attribution assignments for the risk adjusted mortality and complications rates and creates a schedule to review the remaining indicator attributions over the next few months.

Lessons learned: As data moves from case review to aggregate forms of physician performance measurement, there is often a tendency to assume that there are well-defined systems for physician attribution inherent in the data collection process or software. Medical staffs are often unaware that national data collection systems were designed for looking at the hospital's performance, not individual physician performance. Physician attribution choices have been made internally without the medical staff's involvement. Typically, questions arise once individual level data is distributed to the physicians.

It is also not uncommon for these choices to be communicated verbally among the data abstracting staff. The practice of obtaining a written list of attributions for review by the peer review committee will force a greater degree of rigor in the process and engage the medical staff. By not restricting its concern to the core measures that initially raised the concern, this committee established the principle that all attribution decisions need to evaluated by the medical staff.

Evaluating OPPE Data: Using Benchmarks and Targets for FPPE and the Pursuit of Excellence

The goals of a physician competency report are to provide systematic and timely feedback to the physician and to link the report's finding to the credentialing and privileging process. Both of these goals require a clear understanding of how the data will be interpreted and how physician leaders and the physician receiving the data will use it. Data interpretation is also a critical step in performing effective ongoing professional practice evaluation (OPPE) and in linking OPPE to focused professional practice evaluation (FPPE). How this is done can have either a positive or negative effect on creating a physician performance improvement culture.

The most pressing concern on physicians' minds is the second issue, the use of the data, as discussed in Chapter 8. Data interpretation is mainly an issue of fairness. In a practical sense, fairness is implemented through consistency of interpretation and transparency of how the data will be interpreted.

For example, physicians feel a process is fair if the data is interpreted the same way by whoever happens to be the department chair that year. Physicians also feel the process is fair if the basis for interpretation is known in advance. This approach requires medical staff–determined prospective targets. Physician leaders must define how the data will be interpreted before data are distributed to ensure a successful competency report that provides feedback and is fairly integrated into the credentialing process.

Two terms need to be defined for the purpose of this book: benchmark and target.

A benchmark is a source of data that places the performance for an indicator into the context of how well others are doing for the same measure. Thus, a benchmark simply provides a description of the field.

A target is a predetermined threshold upon which the evaluation of the data is based. A target, therefore, is a cultural choice made by the evaluating group, like a medical staff, as what actually constitutes good or poor performance based on the group's goals and priorities.

Understanding Normative Data

One source of benchmarking data that can be used to interpret data more fairly is normative data. Here, the individual's data is compared to a group to put the individual performance into context. Comparison in some way to the average or "norm" of the group is the common method. Typically this is done by expressing the data as a percentile rank or relative to a standard deviation from the mean. Both outcomes, like severity-adjusted mortality, and processes, like compliance with core measures, are often evaluated by comparison with the norm.

External normative large-scale databases include data submitted by many organizations. The combined information is used to create a broader benchmark comparison. Examples include state and federal electronic claims databases, regulatory required–measure databases, hospital consortiums, vendor-specific customer databases, and specialty society-specific databases.

The power of benchmarking with normative data is twofold: 1) it shows all levels of performance so excellent physicians are identified as well as those in need of improvement and 2) since the group norm moves as the group improves as a whole, using normative comparisons drives the pursuit of excellence. Figure 9.1 further illustrates the use of normative data.

The key issue with normative data is what group will be used to establish the norm. While many medical staffs will provide physicians with the average performance for their department or for the medical staff as a whole, this is generally a relatively small group and lacks the perspective of how the rest of the world is doing. Cardiovascular surgery programs that participate in large-scale databases, such as the Society of Thoracic Surgeons database, will have much better normative data than the programs that just use internal comparisons. However, participation in these normative groups often requires commitment of additional resources for the software and abstracting personnel.

Unfortunately, normative data is often not available today for some of the indicators we would like to measure. This is often due to medical staff's desire to make a performance measure so customized to its own organization that it precludes other organizations from obtaining comparison data. As we will discuss about setting targets, a key principle to keep in mind is that it is better to use an imperfect indicator that can be interpreted more fairly through normative data than a perfect one, which can only use internal data to interpret.

EVALUATING OPPE DATA: USING BENCHMARKS AND TARGETS FOR FPPE AND THE PURSUIT OF EXCELLENCE

9.1 Understanding and Using Normative Data

Normative data is data that provides a comparison with some defined group to create an understanding of what is the middle, or norm, of the group. In contrast to comparison with an absolute standard, this allows an individual or organization to see where it ranks relative to the others in that group. The two main reasons for using normative data are that it recognizes all levels of performance and it moves with improvement in the field.

The first step in using normative data is to understand the best way to measure the middle of the group. There are three measures of the norm that are called measures of central tendency: the mean (the average value), the median (the middle value), and the mode (the most frequent value). Which one you use greatly depends on the distribution of the data within a given group.

If the distribution is "normal" (i.e., a classic symmetrical bell-shaped curve, shown below as normal distribution), then all three of these measures result in the same value. However, if the distribution is skewed (i.e. not symmetrical, shown below as skewed distribution), so there are more extreme values on one end of the curve than the other, then the mean, median, and mode will be different. The mean is the most greatly affected by a skewed distribution while the median, otherwise called the 50th percentile, is much less affected. Since most healthcare performance data are skewed, using the median is the best way to measure where the center or middle of the group is located.

**Bell-shaped vs. Skewed distributions:
Effect on Mean, Median and Mode**

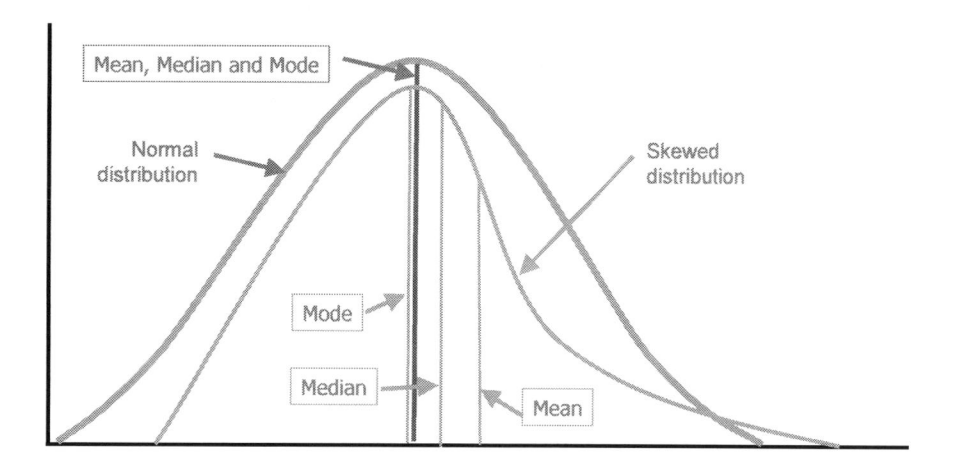

> ### 9.1 Understanding and Using Normative Data (cont.)
>
> The second step in using normative data is to understand the best way to analyze and express the data. Just as the medium was less affected by outliers in a skewed distribution, using percentile rank rather than absolute data values helps to understand how the individual or organization's performance compares to the rest of the field. This can be expressed by the exact percentile rank for a given value (e.g., the 87th percentile) or in which quartile the value was located (e.g., the top 25th percentile). This way, if you improve faster than the group, you will recognize your progress. Similarly, if the field improves over time, you will be aware of whether you are keeping up with the group.
>
> Normative data is not perfect. It can clearly be affected by what group you are being compared to and how the members of the group were chosen. For example, if hospitals are being compared for mortality rates, does the comparison group include all hospitals or ones with specific characteristics (e.g., size, academic programs, etc.)? Asking questions about the composition of your normative group is critical to data interpretation and acceptance.

Interpreting OPPE Data for a Time Interval

OPPE requires having aggregate data on physician performance at regular intervals. The key question is, "How do you interpret that data?" You can analyze aggregate performance data in two ways:

- Use thresholds or targets to interpret overall performance at a particular time interval

- Perform a trend analysis, which looks at variation in performance over time

For either approach, you must define in advance the basis for interpreting the data to achieve good inter-rater reliability. Let's look first at the use of targets to interpret data for a time interval.

Reducing a physician's performance data to a single number over time essentially asks whether the physician's overall performance for that period of time was acceptable. Using this approach, you could review the data every six months as part of OPPE or two years' worth of data at reappointment. This is not the same as identifying a trend, which is noticing a change in performance over time. Note that even when peer review committees "track and trend" individual cases they are often attempting

EVALUATING OPPE DATA: USING BENCHMARKS AND TARGETS FOR FPPE AND THE PURSUIT OF EXCELLENCE

to determine whether the total number of occurrences over time is excessive and necessitates further action. However, without predetermined targets for how many is too many, that approach may be viewed as arbitrary.

The analysis of aggregate data for a defined period of time begins with setting a target for when more detailed analysis is required. Unfortunately, although many medical staffs collect aggregate and comparative data, they stop short of setting an acceptable level of performance. Though these medical staffs may include the department or hospital average with the individual's data, they fail to set a target to ensure that the physician and the physician leader interpret the data in the same manner.

For example, imagine an OPPE profile at appointment that shows that a physician's mortality rate is higher than the department average and, unfortunately, there is no predefined level of what is too high to trigger further investigation. In addition, the committee or department chair must decide what to do at the worst possible time—at reappointment—when he or she knows the decision will affect a specific physician. This lack of clear targets makes it all too easy to say, "Let's give it another few months."

The way to address this problem is simple: Set targets for how to interpret every rule and rate indicator before collecting and reviewing the data. Setting performance expectations in advance of measurement and feedback is only fair, as noted in the discussion of the performance pyramid in Chapter 2. Targets provide physicians with inter-rater reliability for interpreting the data, are more efficient because committee members don't have to debate whether further analysis is required, and are therefore fairer to physicians.

Exceeding a target threshold does not mean a corrective action is required. It simply triggers the question "Why are you different?" Setting these targets in advance requires the medical staff to be actively involved in the indicator selection process and to exercise discipline by determining a reasonable target before the data quality staff sends the data to the committee.

Setting targets prospectively has another advantage for implementing both OPPE and FPPE. Targets make it easier for department chairs to scan the OPPE reports to ensure that no action is needed because the data is within the target range. Targets let you know that a more detailed assessment of the data is needed (FPPE) so that potential performance issues can be addressed in a timely manner.

To achieve a culture focused on improving physician performance, set two targets for each rule or rate indicator. One target is for acceptable performance and the other target is for excellent performance. This approach goes back to the bad apples discussion in Chapter 2: If the only target is acceptable performance, all medical staff members that meet that criterion are considered to be at the same performance level, which clearly is not the case. Setting two targets creates three performance levels:

- Excellent
- Acceptable
- Needs follow-up

This approach recognizes physicians who are performing at a higher level and stimulates those in the middle to pursue excellence. Recognizing excellence in performance can have a profound effect on your medical staff culture and only takes little extra time to perform by setting the targets for excellence.

How to Set Indicator Targets

When setting targets, three questions are usually asked:

- Which indicators need targets?
- Where do you get the targets?
- Who should set the targets?

Which indicators need targets?

Targets are needed for indicators that result in aggregation of the data, which means that each rule and rate indicator needs a target. Individual case review indicators or criteria do not need a target because each case is analyzed and the appropriateness of care is determined. However, for OPPE you should set a target for the aggregate number of cases that were reviewed resulting in specific rating (e.g., significant improvement opportunity) over a particular period.

Where do you get the targets?

The traditional means of obtaining targets was through reviewing literature on a specific issue. Literature benchmark data can be useful because it uses a definition of good performance from outside the hospital. There are two caveats, however, to using literature-based targets: 1) the literature may not measure precisely the same indicator that you are measuring and 2) the literature may not reflect current practice if the clinical practice is undergoing substantial changes. In our current healthcare environment of rapid change, this often makes literature-based benchmarks out of date by the time they are published.

National benchmarking normative databases are the best source to turn to when setting targets. These databases overcome the limitations of literature because the measures are exactly the same and the data are collected continuously, so the benchmark will change as the field changes.

Severity- and risk-adjusted normative data provide the best form of normative benchmark data for setting targets when gathering outcomes data. These data are derived from large-scale normative databases in which statistically determined adjustments have been made to the measured outcomes by evaluating the factors that contribute to a patient's severity of illness or risk. Obtaining normative benchmarking data will take time and resources.

Unfortunately, national benchmarks are not available for every indicator you need to measure. In such circumstances, other options are to use either historical data or consensus-based perceived standards.

Hospital or department historical data allow a normative group comparison approach, but because the group size tends to be small, the perspective is limited. Moreover, using only internal data means that half of the physicians are below average and the other half are above average, which can result in inappropriate follow-up of well-performing physicians in the bottom half or a false sense of good performance in the top half. Still, internal data is better than no data at all for setting an initial target if external data is unavailable.

The last method for target setting is using consensus-based perceived standards. This is where a group (such as the peer review committee) defines the target and the individuals under review (the medical staff) accept the target as reasonable. This approach should be used when there are no other options, such as when an indicator is just starting to be measured. Obtaining some "quick and dirty" data helps determine whether perception was in the ballpark.

Since there tend to be no external benchmarks for rule indicators, using consensus-based targets is a reasonable starting point. Figure 9.2 provides examples of rule indicators for each dimension of physician performance.

9.2 Sample Rule Indicators and Targets

Performance dimension	Excellence target	Acceptable target
Clinical quality		
Blood product use not meeting criteria	1	4
Heparin protocol not used for patient prescribed heparin	0	2
Service quality		
ED page response w/in 30 minutes	1	4
Incidents of delayed consultation	0	2
Validated patient complaints on physician communication/responsiveness	0	3
Patient safety		
Incidents of illegible medication orders	2	4
Incidents of non-participation in pre-procedure timeouts	0	1
H&P not dictated within 24 hrs	0	2
Resource use		
Delayed starts in OR/procedure area	1	4
ICU patients meeting discharge criteria not discharged when requested by medical director	0	3
Physician's discharge instructions not completed at time when patient ready for discharge	1	5
Peer and coworker relationships		
Validated physician behavior Incidents	0	3
Citizenship		
Medical records suspensions	0	3

Even though normative benchmarking data may not be available for many physician performance measures, don't let that prevent you from setting reasonable targets as a starting point and then using your experience to validate whether the targets are appropriate.

For example, if a local target was set too low and the majority of physicians are outside the acceptable range, further investigation will show that either the practice really was acceptable and the target needs adjustment or there is a general problem that needs a broader solution. On the other hand, if a local target is set too high and no one is ever outside the acceptable level, either the indicator is unnecessary or the target needs to be revisited. Treating targets as adjustable based on experience will help the medical staff initially accept them as a work in progress.

EVALUATING OPPE DATA: USING BENCHMARKS AND TARGETS FOR FPPE AND THE PURSUIT OF EXCELLENCE

Who should set the targets?

Physician competency reports evaluate physician performance. Therefore, it is critical that the medical staff determines the targets for excellent and acceptable performance. To ensure medical staff participation in this process, the medical staff quality committee should ask each medical staff department for recommendations for specialty-specific indicators. The quality committee should then establish non-specialty-related measures (e.g., appropriateness of blood product use or patient complaints). The committee should then send these recommendations to the medical executive committee for approval.

By following this process, medical staff leaders will be able to explain to physicians who fall outside established targets and who challenge those targets that the medical staff determined the targets—not the quality office or administration. Again, it is critical that targets are set prior to distributing and interpreting competency reports. Further, targets should be reviewed regularly (e.g., at least annually) to ensure that they are up to date.

No matter what type of benchmark data is used, targets must be set for excellent and acceptable performance. For example, the administration may decide that it would like to be at the 90th percentile of national measures for congestive heart failure. The medical staff still needs to decide what is considered to be excellent performance and what is considered to be acceptable performance for an individual physician. One medical staff might define excellent performance as better than the 90th percentile in a national normative database and acceptable performance as better than the 50th percentile. Another medical staff may choose to define the excellent and acceptable targets as the 75th and 25th percentiles, respectively.

Targets for Indicator Types

Setting targets for review, rate, and rule indicators differ because of the nature of each indicator type. Review and rule indicators are based on a number of events therefore the target must reflect a number, while rate indicators have a denominator and, therefore, may be expressed in a variety of ways.

Review indicator targets

As mentioned earlier, individual review indicators don't need targets because every case is reviewed in-depth. However, for OPPE it is appropriate to set targets for the number of cases in which care is scored for a given rating over a specified period of time. In essence, doing so creates a rule for the number of cases with that rating that are considered unusual for your medical staff and that would trigger more intensive follow-up through FPPE. The following targets are typically used:

- Excellent performance = Zero cases rated care significant improvement opportunity for 12 months

- Acceptable performance = Fewer than three cases rated care significant improvement opportunity for 12 months

Although some medical staffs use a target for the number of cases sent for review, or for the number of cases rated "care appropriate," I don't recommend it because that is more likely to depend on the criteria for review and physician volume. If a physician has a large number of cases coming to review but care is never determined to have improvement opportunities, either the review indicators are too broad, some of the review indicators should be converted to rate measures, or the committee is not doing its job identifying less-than-appropriate care.

Rule indicator targets

Rule indicator targets should reflect the number of times the physician's performance fell outside the target over a set period. Remember, the physician still gets automatic feedback via an educational letter each time the rule is not complied with. However, until the acceptable threshold is exceeded, there is no need for further dialogue or action with the physician.

When setting rule indicator targets, keep in mind that the more critical it is for physicians to comply with the rule, the lower the target levels should be for excellent and acceptable performance. For example, less critical clinical rules such as "No transfusion of red blood cells where hemoglobin is greater than 7 grams unless there is active bleeding or the patient is medically unstable" typically have the following targets:

- Excellent performance = Fewer than two incidents for 12 months

- Acceptable performance = Fewer than four incidents for 12 months

The excellence target conveys the message that even an excellent physician may not meet the criteria once per year. It also indicates that there is no need for intensive follow-up if the physician does not meet the criteria only three times per year. Such targets save a great deal of committee discussion time justifying individual transfusion cases. However, as discussed earlier, targets are a culture choice. If your medical staff has excellent blood usage, you may choose lower targets for excellent or acceptable performance.

Highly critical safety rules such as "Participation in pre-procedure timeout" require lower targets, typically:

- Excellent performance = Zero incidents for 12 months

- Acceptable performance = Fewer than two incidents for 12 months

The excellence target is set at zero because this rule is a national safety standard and the vast majority of physicians now comply with it. The acceptable target is set at fewer than two incidents per year because this rule is so important that if a physician doesn't self-correct after the first educational letter is sent, more intensive follow-up is needed.

Rate indicator targets

You can often find benchmark data for rate indicator targets. However, you can express rate data in two main ways:

1. As an absolute value, such as 23% or 5.3 days

2. As a relative value, such as the 75th percentile or as a statistically defined outlier (e.g., plus or minus 1 standard deviation from the mean) or a ratio (e.g., actual outcomes divided by expected outcomes)

And of course, the target needs to be expressed in the same measurement format as the indicator—it is not uncommon for physician profiles to accidentally show the indicator data expressed as percentages but the targets as percentiles.

Although absolute values are easier to use, relative values work better to drive performance improvement because they allow performance expectations to change as the group norm changes without having to revise the target every year. Some organizations express the target as an absolute value for ease of understanding, but they select that value using a statistically determined formula. For example, the excellence target for surgical complications could be an absolute, such as 1.3%, but that number would be selected each year by a rule that determines the value for physicians at the 75th percentile of a national database.

When external data aren't available for rate measures and targets need to be selected based on internal data, using historical data and setting targets based on the mean and the distribution of that data is the best approach. For internal data, using percentiles is less useful because it guarantees that in a department of 10 physicians, two will be below the 25th percentile, even if their performance is very close to that of others on the distribution.

Interpreting OPPE Data for Trends

There are two ways to look for a trend. The first is to look for changes in the point-in-time categorical ratings. The second is to use formal trend analysis tools.

Defining trends by changes in categorical ratings

A simple, practical method for determining a trend is to follow the categorical rating of excellent, acceptable, and needs follow-up for each indicator over time and define a rule for when a trend occurs. In Chapter 10, we will discuss the options for defining an OPPE trend using this approach and show an example of a categorical trend report in Chapter 11.

How often should rate and rule aggregate data be reviewed? The Joint Commission at this time requires at least three evaluations in a two-year reappointment cycle. For those who wish to stick to the minimum, that means producing an OPPE report every eight months. However, I recommend creating reports every six months for three reasons:

1. It is more aligned with the typical quality and financial data availability cycles in most organizations

2. It allows for chances for feedback in the two-year reappointment cycle and hence, a greater opportunity for physician self-improvement

3. Because it provides more frequent categorical ratings, it is easier to identify a trend sooner for elevation to FPPE

Beyond what The Joint Commission recommends, organizations still often ask, "How often is enough?" (i.e., how often would you recommend?) Two issues affect the answer. The first issue is whether the frequency evaluated will produce interpretable data on an individual physician level. As the reporting frequency increases, if the data is based only on that time period, the numbers will get

EVALUATING OPPE DATA: USING BENCHMARKS AND TARGETS FOR FPPE AND THE PURSUIT OF EXCELLENCE

smaller and less interpretable. For that reason I recommend using a rolling data time period that makes sense no matter what the frequency of the OPPE report.

For example, mortality due to heart failure, while a relatively frequent occurrence for the hospital as a whole on a six-month basis, would have few physicians with sufficient numbers of cases for interpretation at that frequency. Using a rolling 12 months, or even a rolling two years of data for each OPPE report, would provide a more accurate interpretation of physician performance.

The second issue is how much of a burden producing and reviewing reports for OPPE puts on your quality staff and department chairs. Obviously, the more frequent the reporting, the greater the burden. For those organizations that have decision support tools where physicians can access their data at any time, one might think this issue would go away. However, OPPE doesn't just involve the physician reviewing his or her own data; members of the medical staff also must look at it. Thus, there is still the issue of the burden for review by the department chair and the follow-up activities for the quality staff.

Analyzing variation in performance with formal tools

Variation analysis, also called trend analysis, can be conducted using more formal tools like run charts and control charts. Among other things, these charts can identify when performance falls above or below a predetermined target or when a data pattern violates defined rules of random variation. Any in-depth discussion of how to analyze variation over time is beyond the scope of this book for physician competency reports.

This approach is most useful if the indicator is of a high-enough volume that variations are statistically significant. Thus, it is usually not a good tool for routinely following physician performance measures at the individual physician level for OPPE. However, control charts and run charts are very useful when looking at data for the whole medical staff or for a specific group of physicians. It also can be useful as a secondary analysis tool when an initial target is exceeded for individual physicians with reasonably high-volume indicators or when there is a need for FFPE monitoring to look for improvement.

10 From OPPE to FPPE: Creating Accountability for Physician Performance Improvement

When the evaluation of data indicates a potential improvement opportunity, the ongoing professional practice evaluation (OPPE) process moves to a more focused evaluation of the physician's performance, and if the data warrants it, identification and implementation of improvement opportunities. This process is called focused professional practice evaluation (FPPE). In one sense, there is nothing new about the concept that inadequate performance needs to be addressed; the case review process has traditionally had this step in place. What is new is that the review of aggregate data also needs a process to effectively address improvement opportunities. This was the primary impact of The Joint Commission requirements of OPPE and FPPE.

As was discussed in Chapter 2, peer review can be done punitively or positively and still meet the regulatory requirements. The goal of this chapter is to provide an approach that will create a performance improvement culture while maintaining the leadership accountabilities needed to address physician performance concerns.

Let's begin by asking the question, "At what levels of the physician performance pyramid are OPPE and FPPE?" OPPE is a starting point for identifying improvement opportunities. This can be based on a single serious or egregious incident or a failure to meet targets on aggregate data. This activity falls in the pyramid level of measuring physician performance.

You might think FPPE begins when an improvement plan is created (the managing poor performance pyramid level); however, in a performance improvement culture, FPPE really has four steps:

1. To confirm whether a physician performance improvement opportunity exists

2. To help determine the root cause that will help the physician improve

3. To create an improvement plan to address the cause

4. To monitor the plan to determine whether performance is improved

With steps 1 and 2, FPPE actually begins at the performance feedback level of the pyramid when a leader reviews outlier data with a physician to determine why the physician is different. When this occurs, the OPPE process has gone beyond just providing feedback for self-improvement. The need for further explanation or "drill down" is important to identify whether the data is accurate and a real improvement opportunity exists. If the data turns out to be inaccurate and no improvement opportunity exists, the FPPE process would stop at this level.

When an opportunity is found, FPPE moves up the pyramid to the managing physician performance level through steps 3 and 4. Here informal or formal improvement plans are developed to guide the FPPE process. This is that part of FPPE that is much less comfortable for many physician leaders; there needs to be clear policies and procedures to maintain accountability for both the physician under the FPPE plan and the leaders who created it.

An important feature of FPPE in a performance improvement culture is to make sure FPPE is not considered an "investigation" or adverse action in your medical staff bylaws. An investigation should be defined as when the medical executive committee (MEC) is considering formal restriction of privileges or membership. This way, FPPE is not reportable to the National Practitioner Data Bank or to most state agencies. By treating FPPE as a step below these actions, it allows for more cooperative participation by the physicians in addressing improvement opportunities and reflects the cultural value of seeking physician improvement first.

Accountability for FPPE Initiation, Monitoring, and Follow-Up

As discussed in Chapter 9, determining the need for initiating FPPE from OPPE data is best performed by evaluating physician performance against predetermined targets. How this is done should be defined in your peer review policy. Most organizations assume this must occur whenever there is an outlier on any indicator, but this is not always the case. For example, some organizations will require follow-up when the indicator data falls below acceptable targets for two sequential time periods. This approach allows for physician improvement and reduces the burden of department chairs following up on isolated indicator results.

Generally, the peer review committee or the MEC are the bodies that oversee the FPPE process. While either mechanism is acceptable from a regulatory standpoint, in an improvement focused culture, FPPE works best if it is kept below the MEC level so it is not confused with an investigation. Having the peer review committee work collaboratively with the department chairs to manage and monitor

FROM OPPE TO FPPE: CREATING ACCOUNTABILITY FOR PHYSICIAN PERFORMANCE IMPROVEMENT

FPPE lowers the anxiety level that a physician's privileges are in imminent danger and focuses more on successfully completing the improvement cycle. Of course, the peer review committee reports to the MEC on FPPEs that it is working on, but that is different than the MEC directly overseeing the FPPE process.

Using that approach as a model, what are the respective responsibilities of the peer review committee and the department chairs? Although the relative authority of each group may vary among medical staffs, having both involved in the FPPE process creates a better sense of accountability and fairness. In general, the department chair is the driving force behind FPPE, and the oversight body (typically the peer review committee) plays the role of ensuring department chair accountability and consistency. Often if the organization has a physician executive like a vice president of medical affairs (VPMA) or chief medical officer (CMO), that individual can assist both the committee and the department chairs to meet their responsibilities because they have more training and experience in managing physician performance. However, the responsibilities for FPPE must rest within a medical staff line of authority. Outlined below are the main FPPE functions of the oversight committee and department chairs.

Peer review committee (or MEC if it provides direct oversight) responsibilities:

- Set targets for OPPE data: As discussed in Chapter 9, this provides the basis for minimizing personal bias by the department chairs

- Ensures timely review of OPPE data by department chair: This is accomplished by summary reports to the committee from each department chair regarding the findings of any physicians in need of follow-up for specific indicators

- Approves requests from department chair for initiating FPPE: This provides oversight so that the department chair will not be accused of personal bias in initiating FPPE

- Reviews FPPE plans: This provides a sense of fairness and consistency across departments

- Tracks results of FPPE: If a formal improvement plan is established, the committee should receive regular reports on how the plan is working and a final report and recommendation from the department chair once it is completed

- Report to the MEC (unless the MEC is the oversight body): The goal is not for the MEC to review and take action of each FPPE but to be informed on a regular basis of the following:

- Number and type of improvement opportunities identified

- Improvement plans initiated

- Improvement plans requested from department chairs; plans deemed inadequate or not received

- Implemented improvement plan completion report and recommendations

- Requests for formal investigation or corrective action when needed for improvement plan failures

Department chair responsibilities:

- Reviews OPPE data and determines reasons for outliers: This can be done either as a formal or informal process with the physician, as described in the next section

- Determines the need for FPPE: This should be done through a recommendation to the appropriate peer review committee

- Develops the FPPE plan: This can be accomplished with assistance if requested from the committee chair, VPMA, and quality staff

- Monitors FPPE results for improvement: This includes both an evaluation of the results and a recommendation to the committee on next steps if not completed successfully

- Evaluates FPPE results in credentialing/privileging recommendations to the credentials committee: This provides the link between FPPE and the credentialing and privileging process

Designing an Effective FPPE Plan

Often physicians are asked to create an improvement plan without clear guidance as to what it should include. A poorly developed improvement plan is a disservice to both the physician under the FPPE and for the medical staff when trying to evaluate the results. To be effective, improvement plans need to begin with the end in mind by providing clear measurable goals and a method for obtaining the data needed to evaluate its success. The principles are the same as any standard quality improvement method. Outlined below is an example of the elements of a good FPPE plan:

- Improvement action: What will the physician do differently based on the improvement opportunity defined by the OPPE data?

- Improvement goal/milestones: What degree of change is expected in the data overall and, if appropriate, what interim milestones will demonstrate that the improvement has begun and is progressing?

- Time frames for achieving goal/milestones: When are the goal and any interim milestones expected to be achieved?

- Method of monitoring: Is monitoring the OPPE data sufficient or will additional data collection specific to the improvement opportunity be needed to demonstrate improvement?

- Next steps if goals are not achieved: What will be the anticipated consequences for the physician if the FPPE goal is not met?

The last component is one that is often avoided by physician leaders who wish to be collegial and feel that describing consequences this early in the process would be detrimental to that value. However, not including this element is actually unfair to the physician and creates political gridlock when the physician cries out to the medical staff, "You never told me that it would come to this!" The consequences at this stage do not have to be precise but can provide more of a general guidance such as a second round of monitoring, shortened or conditional renewal of privileges, or request to the MEC to consider formal action.

Getting Physician Buy-In for Improvement Opportunities and FPPE

When individual physicians demonstrate poor clinical performance and have been unable to improve that performance on their own, medical staff leaders must step in and manage the situation. To the extent that it is possible, such an intervention should be both systematic and timely.

The old saying "It takes two to tango" comes to mind when discussing working with physicians on FPPE. A tango is best performed by partners working together in harmony. Similarly, in a performance improvement culture, if the department chair and the physician with the improvement opportunity can work together, the result will be more satisfying for both parties.

CHAPTER 10

The first step of working together requires the buy-in of the physician that indeed an improvement opportunity exists. This is greatly affected by your current medical staff culture. If your current culture is viewed as positive, this is not a difficult process. However, if it is viewed as punitive or if the physician has not yet bought into the culture values of improvement, the response to an improvement opportunity is likely to be defensive.

So how do you overcome this defensive posture? It begins with how the physician is informed of the potential opportunity. For FPPE that is based on OPPE data, the physician should be aware of the issue by receiving his or her OPPE report at the same time as the department chair. Then the department chair follow-up can begin with, "Because your OPPE report for this indicator was outside the target for two data periods in a row, per the medical staff policy, we need to discuss why this might be occurring." If the OPPE reports are not routinely distributed to the physician, the department chair's task is more difficult because the department chair must explain what the data shows.

Once the physician is aware of the need to discuss the data, the nature of the initial interaction should be open-minded and collegial with the goal of defining the actual improvement opportunity or determining that more data is needed. This step should include an effort to mutually develop a differential diagnosis as to the causative factors such as knowledge deficit, technical deficiency, poor judgment, documentation deficiencies, or communication failures.

Once an opportunity is defined, the approach for further interactions should be determined by the level of concern. This is a judgment call on the part of the department chair and the appropriate peer review committee. For indicators that are not critical or for first-time issues, an informal meeting may be sufficient. For more serious issues, a formal process may be needed. The critical step in either situation is establishing whether the physician accepts ownership of the improvement opportunity. The box below outlines a typical process for both the informal and formal approaches.

In planning your approach, know what your goals are and where the focus should be. Ask yourself, who will be at the meeting? It may be one-on-one between the physician and department chair, or it may be necessary to involve other people. Where will the meeting take place? If collegial, the meeting may occur at the physician's office or a neutral site. The more formal proceedings typically take place at the department chair's office. Finally, when will the meeting take place, and what are the established timelines for it?

As department chair, it is wise to practice your approach, particularly if you do not have extensive experience in this area. During the meeting, you will want to reference your role and stress to the physician that it is not a personal situation. Describe the concern in a non-judgmental manner, and state your goal for the session. Expect resistance from the physician in most cases, and be prepared to maintain consistency of position and purpose in the face of it. Ultimately, the goal is to achieve an agreed-upon action plan of performance improvement.

What Happens if FPPE Fails?

Of course, if a physician is unwilling or unable to improve, there may be no choice but to proceed to the last level of the pyramid, taking corrective action. Also, if the issues at hand are thought to put patients at immediate risk, going directly to summary suspension and following your bylaws to resolve those concerns is required.

In either case, the leader must know its organization's bylaws and be certain to follow them strictly. Early consultation with legal counsel in potentially problematic situations is also encouraged. Ultimately, a formal investigation may have to be initiated, and external peer review should be considered, if it has not already been used.

DEPARTMENT CHAIR–PHYSICIAN INTERACTIONS FOR OPPE DATA

Informal approach

- Discuss potential causes for outlier status (determine whether additional data are needed)
    - If physician owns cause, discuss potential improvement actions by the physician
    - If the physician does not accept ownership of the cause, consider obtaining additional influential medical staff leadership involvement or moving to the formal approach

- Obtain verbal commitment to the physician improvement actions

- Memorialize cause and improvement action commitment in a memo (does not need to go in the physician's file)

- No further action/specific monitoring unless recurrence (e.g., OPPE data does not improve)

Formal approach

- Discuss potential causes for outlier status (determine whether additional data are needed)

CHAPTER 10

> **DEPARTMENT CHAIR–PHYSICIAN INTERACTIONS FOR OPPE DATA (CONT.)**
>
> - Define specific improvement actions to be implemented by the physician
>
> - Create draft FPPE plan
>
> - Obtain written commitment from the physician to the FPPE plan
>   - If physician will not commit to the plan, consider obtaining additional influential leadership involvement or report back to the oversight body and allow them to determine next steps
>
> - Monitor FPPE results for improvement
>
> - Meet with the physician at predetermined milestones and document progress or communication of next steps

FPPE for New Members and Privileges: Why Is It Different?

As noted in Chapter 1, the process for performing FPPE that is part of the initial credentialing and privileging process or for new privilege requests is not covered in this book. However, it is important to briefly note why this process of FFPE differs from the FPPE process described in this chapter.

First, this use of FPPE begins with a routine monitoring process, not with a concern. This monitoring generally combines audits or observations of selected cases that represent samples related to the physician's requested privileges and more timely review of OPPE data. Thus, when doing this FPPE one does not start with the question "Why are you different?" The question here is: "Does the information you provided to attest to your competency match what we observe in our setting?" Hopefully, if the department chair and credentials committee have done a good job, the answer will be yes.

Second, since this process is more directly tied to privileging decisions made by the credentials committee, it is more typical that the credentials committee oversees this component of FPPE. This will ensure that if issues are identified early in the course of a physician exercising privileges, it can be addressed in a timely fashion.

Case Study: Initiating an FPPE for Mortality Data

Scenario: In January, the hospital implemented a new severity-adjusted software program for mortality data based on electronic claims information. The quality management staff provided the peer review committee (PRC) with an initial presentation describing the data system and requested that the data be distributed to the medical staff with the data attributed to the attending physician. The initial discussion focused on starting with a few diagnosis-related groups that would be more likely to have mortality as an expected outcome.

In February, the PRC authorized the distribution of data for congestive heart failure (CHF). The data was to be expressed as an index of actual deaths divided by expected deaths. Because the overall hospital mortality index for CHF over the past year was 0.95, based on the recommendation of the department of medicine, the targets for individual physician performance evaluation were set at 0.85 for excellent performance and 1.25 for acceptable performance. The PRC requested that the most recent data available be presented at its March meeting, prior to distribution to physicians.

Quality staff members prepared a report for the data from the third quarter of the previous year, the most recent quarter analyzed by the hospital's vendor. The report included all 19 physicians in the department of medicine. Eight of the physicians were specialists in non-cardiac areas and had no CHF patients. Four physicians appeared to exceed the acceptable target. However, most of the internists, including those exceeding the target, had only a few CHF admissions in that quarter.

The quality staff was concerned that using only one quarter's worth of data would make the data difficult to interpret. However, because the data came from electronic claims data, the vendor had analyzed the data for the past four years. The quality staff consulted the PRC chair, who requested that staff members use two years' worth of data to align with the reappointment cycle and eliminate from the report any physicians that had no CHF admissions.

Lesson learned:

- Although quality staff members are often eager to send data to the medical staff, it is wise to have a physician group review the data to be sure it makes sense prior to the initial distribution of data attributed to physicians. This reduces the likelihood of statistical bias due to obvious issues with the data's accuracy.

- While analyzing data quarterly might be useful on a hospital-wide level, using data periods that are too short to accrue sufficient cases for individual physicians usually results in over interpretation. There is no requirement for defining data time periods. Although The Joint Commission's OPPE requires organizations to look at data more frequently (e.g., approximately every six months) than at reappointment, the time period to review data can be a rolling two years. This will help reduce statistical bias based on small numbers.

- If data is not relevant to a physician practice, it should not be used to evaluate performance. If a physician has CHF admissions but no deaths, the data can be used because the opportunity for mortality was present. However, if the physician has no CHF patients, zero mortality is meaningless.

Committee discussion: At the March meeting, the data from the previous two years was presented to the PRC (see Figure 10.1). Physicians were shown by code number to reduce conflict of interest. The surgical representative noted that since internist 003 and 005 had exceeded the acceptable target, the committee should request the medicine department chair initiate an FPPE per the medical staff OPPE/FPPE policy by reviewing each of the deaths for both physicians during the committee meeting. Others felt it would be useful to find out what might be causing these results by checking the coding and attribution accuracy and discussing the data with the physicians. One committee member questioned

10.1 CHF Risk-Adjusted Mortality Data (Past Eight Quarters)

Provider ID	# CHF D/Cs	# Actual deaths	# Expected deaths	Mortality index	Excellent targets	Acceptable targets
001	24	3	3	1.00	0.85	1.25
002	43	12	11	1.09	0.85	1.25
003	52	11	7	1.57	0.85	1.25
004	34	6	5	1.20	0.85	1.25
005	10	2	1	2.00	0.85	1.25
006	16	3	4	0.75	0.85	1.25
007	30	6	8	0.75	0.85	1.25
008	41	11	12	0.92	0.85	1.25
009	25	4	8	0.50	0.85	1.25
Dept. total	**275**	**59**	**59**	**1.00**	0.85	1.25

FROM OPPE TO FPPE: CREATING ACCOUNTABILITY FOR PHYSICIAN PERFORMANCE IMPROVEMENT

whether it was worthwhile to look at physician 005 since there were only 10 patients for the two years and only two deaths, one of which was expected.

The committee decided that the concern about the low volume for physician 005 was legitimate and represented flaws in the OPPE/FPPE policy. It decided to modify the policy and require at least 30 patients or at least four expected deaths be present prior to initiating an FPPE.

Regarding physician 003, since this was the first time the committee was evaluating the mortality data, it decided to first look at the coding and attribution accuracy prior to having the committee and department chairs meet with the physician. Prior to meeting with the physician, the quality staff provided a list of the CHF patients attributed to the physician and the ICD-9 coding, demographic data, and admission location for each patient. This analysis indicated the attribution was reasonably correct but several patients appeared more severely ill than coding described.

The committee and medicine department chairs met with the physician and shared the patient list and the initial data showing the physician's performance relative to the rest of the department. The chairs indicated that this was a new process and they all needed to learn together what the data meant. In general, the meeting was collegial and the physician, although surprised that he was an outlier, indicated he was new to all this and open to suggestions on how to understand and improve the data.

The physician was first asked whether there were any inaccuracies in the patient list or the coding that he noticed. He indicated that at least two of the 52 patients were assigned incorrectly in the database because, although he was the admitting physician, he was not the attending for that case. When reviewing the coding data, the physician commented that he thought several of his patients who were admitted to the ICU had comorbid conditions that were not reflected in the coding. He also indicated that a few of the deaths were terminal nursing home patients whom he had admitted out of courtesy to the family and who died within 24 hours of admission. They also discussed with the physician why a few of the mortalities were admitted directly from home to a routine monitored bed rather than going through the emergency department (ED) for evaluation. The physician replied that he was trying to avoid the ED delays for patients.

Following the meeting, the chair asked the hospital staff to review the coding and administrative issues. The health information management (HIM) director agreed that two of the cases were incorrectly assigned, but because only one of the two cases had been a mortality that was expected, it did not explain the elevated index. She also provided data showing that the physician responded to HIM prompts for better documentation of comorbidities only 50% of the time, compared to 90% for the other internists. The case management director indicated that the physician's use of observation status was below that of the other internists.

Lessons learned:

- Having a private discussion with a physician regarding new types of data is generally more effective than bringing him or her to a committee meeting inquisition.

- To obtain the physician's perspective, start by asking, "Why do you think your mortality rate is different from your colleagues?" It is best to have some preliminary "drill down" detailed data prepared for the common questions such as "Which patients?" "Why were they admitted?" and "What were their diagnoses?"

- Starting with the administrative factors makes the physician feel that you are looking first at competency related to systems and communication rather than attacking his or her clinical practice. It also helps the physician realize which factors affecting the data are within his or her control.

Committee decision/disposition: The PRC chair presented the findings at the April meeting. The chair summarized his view that the elevated heart failure mortality rate for physician 003 appeared more likely to reflect documentation and resource management practices rather than clinical deficiencies. One of the committee members expressed concern that it was still important to help improve the data since it was publicly available for the hospital and might become so for physicians. The committee decided to initiate an FPPE to address these specific issues where the physician was asked to meet informally with HIM and case management and the department chair to discuss mechanisms to increase responses to coding prompts and requests for use of observation status. The physician was also asked to meet with the ED director and the department of medicine chair to decrease the use of direct admissions to the floor.

The committee requested a report from the department chair on the percentage of response to coding prompts, direct admissions, and observation status at three and six months and to review the mortality data from that time period once it became available from the vendor.

FROM OPPE TO FPPE: CREATING ACCOUNTABILITY FOR PHYSICIAN PERFORMANCE IMPROVEMENT

Follow-up and discussion

The PRC decides to use the information on this case for a grand rounds presentation to make physicians more aware of the impact that documentation and observation status can have on data. The physician works with the staff, and his rate of response to prompts for coding and observation status becomes similar to the rest of the staff.

Lessons learned:

- Although the committee could have merely had an informal discussion with the physician, defining an FPPE helps reinforce the need for improvement.

- Remember, this is not a formal investigation at this time, merely a data-based approach to monitoring improvement. Because the physician is cooperative, it can be done collegially.

- Trust but verify. If you have asked for a change in practice or behavior, it is easier and more timely to monitor that change rather than wait for the outcomes data to come back in six to 12 months.

11 OPPE Profiles and Physician Performance Feedback: Practical Principles for Competency Report Design and Distribution

The previous chapters of this book discussed how to select physician performance measures and how to create a culture for using a physician competency report. The goal of this chapter is to take the performance measures you have obtained and put that data into a coherent physician report for both ongoing professional practice evaluation (OPPE) and physician feedback that can be expanded as new measures are added.

Designing a competency report is like a professional decorator picking out wallpaper. A decorator doesn't pick the color just to match the carpet. The wallpaper is part of the room's overall design scheme. The decorator needs to consider the wallpaper's color pattern and how it will interact with the furniture, the carpet, and the room size.

Similarly, effective competency reports aren't just about the format. They are part of a system that will provide information that can be used to understand and address physician performance issues. Therefore, the design process needs to take into account how the reports will either fit into the current medical staff culture or help lead the cultural change toward better use of performance data.

OPPE Profile and Physician Performance Feedback Report: What Is the Difference?

Even though The Joint Commission requires physician performance *evaluation* through OPPE, the accreditor's standards do not explain how to do it and don't require the organization to provide physician *feedback*. Similarly, other accreditors require a process for evaluating physician performance but do not require routine physician feedback.

Yet many medical staff leaders have concluded that it is unfair to evaluate physicians without giving them access to their own data. As we discussed in Chapter 2, without feedback, it is difficult to create a culture of self-improvement, and as a result, physicians may view peer review as secretive and punitive.

So what is the difference between an OPPE report and a physician feedback report? In reality, the two generally should not differ in content or format. The real difference is in systems that are implemented for the timely distribution of the feedback report to the individual physicians and the OPPE report to the medical staff leaders accountable for the data.

There is still great flexibility in creating a feedback report although the information system used to create it may limit your choices. The best strategy is to ensure that the report you create meets the needs of your medical staff or practice group while also meeting applicable Joint Commission standards. Ironically, by setting out to design a competency feedback report, rather than merely creating a physician competency credentialing profile for the medical staff services department files, your medical staff will accomplish both objectives because the credentials profile will be a natural by-product of the feedback report. So, how should you begin?

Design the Report

In many hospitals, the medical services professionals make decisions about the content of physician reports because the medical staff offers little-to-no guidance in the matter. This model of building physician reporting systems must change. If an organization truly wants to measure physician performance, the medical staff, as a self-governing body of physicians, must take ownership of the project and define which measures to use and how to use them. Although it may seem that the report is merely a technical task for the hospital staff to perform, without physician involvement in the design, there will likely be problems with physician acceptance. Therefore, just as it was recommended in Chapter 5 regarding selecting indicators, use a physician-led group for the report design. Typically, it would be either the peer review committee or a separate work group comprised of the appropriate specialties.

One thing to consider is, if the organization has already selected a software program for the OPPE report, do you still need a design group? The answer is definitely yes. First, every software program has capabilities and limitations. Second, some of the design issues discussed below are independent of the software.

Here are four steps that will help the group design your competency feedback report:

- Define the principles for the use of the data

- Create a format that reflects the design principles

- Develop infrastructure and support materials
- Pilot-test your design to be sure it is effective

Define the Principles: 10 Questions to Guide Your Design

As we discussed in Chapter 8, the most critical issue on physicians' minds is how the hospital will use the data. Therefore, it's best to start your design by reaffirming and expanding the principles that guided indicator selection. Here are 10 questions that can guide development of feedback report principles:

1. Why is the report being distributed?
2. What aspects of competency will the report cover?
3. How will the indicators and targets be selected?
4. Which indicators will be linked to credentialing?
5. Who will receive the data?
6. How often will it be distributed?
7. How should the report be interpreted?
8. When will the physicians be held accountable for performance?
9. How will the report follow-up be performed?
10. How will the report be improved?

Although we will provide some common answers for each question for your consideration that reiterate many of the concepts discussed in previous chapters, do not simply adopt these answers. Your group may have different answers for these questions. It is important that you customize the report for your medical staff culture and hospital data systems.

Answering these questions in a concise document can provide the basis for your medical staff policy and procedure regarding feedback reports. It can also be used as an educational tool in the question-and-answer format for your physicians when the report is first introduced. Let's begin by discussing each of these questions.

Why is the report being distributed?

The first step in any project is to clearly define the goal. Based on the culture described in Chapter 2, I suggest the following five goals:

1. To set clear expectations of physician performance for all competency categories

2. To create a medical staff culture that accepts performance data feedback in the spirit of continuous improvement

3. To make physicians aware of areas of excellent performance, as well as areas of improvement opportunities

4. To allow physicians the opportunity to self-improve based on the data provided

5. To meet Joint Commission standards for OPPE

As was discussed in previous chapters, establishing performance measures and explaining them to physicians up front tells them what the organization expects of them. Creating performance feedback reports forces the medical staff to articulate what it is measuring, what it considers "good" performance, and makes clear that physicians will be given an opportunity to improve.

What aspects of competency will the report cover?

Typically, the goal is to provide a single report with measures for each general competency. Some organizations may not be able to gather all the data together in one report, but that doesn't prevent them from collecting and distributing data on all the competencies simultaneously. This provides reinforcement to the physician that all competencies are being measured systematically and provides a more balanced view of performance.

How will the indicators and targets be selected?

As we discussed in Chapters 5 and 6, the medical staff should select indicators and targets with input from the appropriate departments. A statement defining the committee with the specific responsibility and the ongoing process will help to clarify this issue for the medical staff members who raise concerns about the data. It is also important to affirm the desire for validity of the indicators used in the report by stating that only indicators relevant to physician performance will be used.

Which indicators will be linked to credentialing?

Not all performance feedback data need to be used for reappointment. Therefore, the feedback report may contain indicators for feedback purposes only, which will not be used in reappointment decisions. For example, resource data (e.g., lengths of stay [LOS]) could be considered to be economic credentialing for some medical staffs. Although the data should still be provided in the feedback report, it should be clearly labeled as "not for use in reappointment." The medical executive committee should determine which indicators will be used for reappointment decisions.

Who will receive the data?

Although it would be ideal to send a report to every medical staff member, that is not always realistic or even appropriate, particularly for low-volume providers. The design group should decide the general level of activity that would make the report meaningful.

Another issue to keep in mind is that when a physician receives his or her own data, he or she usually wants to know who else has access to that data. By defining this up front, you increase process transparency.

How often will it be distributed?

Because the goal of performance feedback is to allow physicians to improve performance, a physician's access to his or her performance data shouldn't be restricted. To allow for improvement, performance data must be provided systematically and in a timely manner. If the report is only passively available—in other words, physicians can, if they wish, see their data—many physicians may not bother to look at their reports. In addition, The Joint Commission's standards for OPPE require a systematic and timely review of performance data. Fortunately, these two needs can be met in the same way.

The most practical approach is to distribute the report every six months. This provides a physician with four reports in a two-year cycle and gives him or her a reasonable opportunity for improvement during that period if an indicator is outside the acceptable level and meets The Joint Commission's time frame for OPPE.

How should the report be interpreted?

The indicators in the report provide only broad comparisons and are not precise measures of physician competence. As such, the medical staff must recognize data limitations and interpret the data accordingly. There are two sources of interpretation: the physician receiving the data and the medical staff leader reviewing it. The goal is to have the interpretation of each individual be the same. As discussed in Chapter 9, targets provide a common interpretation of the data.

When will the physicians be held accountable for performance?

Many organizations send out the first reports and immediately want to take action on data that is below expectations. It may be unfair to do so for two reasons:

1. The data may not be entirely accurate, and distributing it to the physicians first is a good way to determine whether that is the case

2. If you want to have a culture of improvement, you must give people time to improve

On the other hand, there are organizations that don't want to distribute the reports until the data are perfect because they want to change their culture into one that accepts data before they it send out. Don't wait for the culture to change before distributing feedback reports. Distributing the reports is part of changing the culture.

Consider using an initial grace period in which reports are distributed but no actions are taken to allow physicians time to understand the data. The grace period may range from six to 12 months depending on how unfamiliar the particular indicator is to the medical staff and should also apply to any new indicators added to the report over time.

How will the report follow-up be performed?

Medical staff leaders must ensure that the physician and the physician leaders are using the reports appropriately. In general, I recommend that the department chair perform the actual follow-up and that a medical staff committee (i.e., peer review committee or medical executive committee) hold the chair accountable to do so. The design group needs to decide when follow-up should occur (e.g., if any single indicator is below the acceptable level, or if two reporting periods in a row are below acceptable). The group also needs to define what is expected of the individual or committee responsible for follow-up in terms of discussion and documentation.

How will the report be improved?

No report will be perfect, especially the first one. The design group must define the process to improve the report over time and define who is responsible for making those improvements.

Create a Format That Reflects the Design Principles

As stated in an earlier chapter, famous architect Louis Sullivan defined the building design principle of "form follows function." That is also true for feedback reports. Applying the aforementioned principles that your design group has defined will help to create a format that reflects those principles. I have found the following four aspects of creating the right format for your report to be helpful:

1. How will the data be organized?

2. How will the data be reported?

3. How will the data be interpreted?

4. How will the data be understood?

How will the data be organized?

To some extent, data organization will be affected by the software program used for the reports. At this stage, if your organization already has a software program, it is important to examine its limitations and capabilities to determine how it affects your design and whether it is adequate for your needs. If you have not yet automated the reports via a software program, this is the time to begin to evaluate the options for your organization. At the end of this chapter we will discuss some common software challenges and solutions.

Organize indicators by core competency

If possible, organize indicators by the physician competence category being measured. This helps physicians understand which competency an indicator measures. This also allows for the interpretation of patterns within a competency, and it demonstrates to The Joint Commission your use of a comprehensive framework to evaluate physician performance.

Although organizing by competency may seem obvious, many hospitals currently organize data in reports by disease (e.g., pneumonia mortality, complications, cost, LOS, and pneumonia core measures). The intent of this approach is to show a physician the extent of his or her success in treating pneumonia patients.

It's more meaningful, however, to organize data by the general competencies. The aim of this approach is to move the conversation away from how well the physician cares for pneumonia patients in general and instead to focus on overall patient care.

For example, organizing the data by competency would place the pneumonia outcomes in the patient care category with other disease outcomes, the resource outcomes in the systems-based practice category with other resource measures, and the core measures in the medical knowledge category with other evidence-based medicine practices. This is more meaningful for defining and interpreting a performance issue pattern. For example, if multiple measures in the medical knowledge category showed poor performance, the focus of the discussion with the physician would be on why the physician is struggling with using evidence-based medicine measures consistently, not just on pneumonia practices.

Separate activity from performance

Physician activity data (i.e., volume data) should be separated from performance data so as not to give the illusion that the hospital is evaluating activity. Activity data describes how much work (e.g., admissions, procedures, or image interpretations) a physician completes within a given period. Performance data, on the other hand, indicates how well a physician does his or her work (e.g., outcomes or patient satisfaction ratings). Hospitals sometimes lump the two together, but doing so isn't very useful. For example, the number of deliveries an obstetrician performs per year doesn't indicate much about the quality of those deliveries.

If you are not sure if an indicator measures activity or performance, set a target as a guide. If you can't set a target for acceptable performance, you shouldn't use it as a performance indicator.

How will the data be reported?

This question asks how you will report the provider's actual data. Although it may seem obvious, you can report the data in a number of ways. Here are some of the key considerations.

Indicator type

Before they look at their own data, physicians need to know whether they are dealing with a review, rate, or rule indicator. Putting this in a column next to the indicator on the feedback report reminds the physician why the data is expressed the way it is shown. For example, rule indicators are expressed as a number of events and they don't have a denominator, whereas rate indicators have a denominator of some type to adjust for volume.

OPPE PROFILES AND PHYSICIAN PERFORMANCE FEEDBACK

Actual data expression

The column with the actual data expression will include different types of data. As mentioned earlier, rule indicators only need to show a number. Rate indicators, on the other hand, can be expressed in a number of ways (e.g., percentage, percentile, average, index). It is important that the numerical format of how the data are expressed is the same as the target format. For example, using percentages for the provider data and percentiles for the target makes the data impossible to interpret. The important concept is to always show the calculated value in the data expression column that will relate to the target. If you show just the raw numbers, the physician is forced to mentally calculate the rate, and it is difficult to relate the data to the target.

In addition to the calculated value, for rate indicators, some organizations like to show both the numerator and the denominator that created the rate as separate columns so that the data can be better understood in relation to the volume of activity. For example, a complication rate of 50% is not meaningful if the numerator is 1 and the denominator is 2 compared to a report in which the numerator is 10 and the denominator is 20. Others may show only the denominator or volume. When dealing with a severity-adjusted index (e.g., actual mortalities/expected mortalities), often both numbers will be shown.

How will the data be interpreted?

This question asks what the rest of the columns in your report will look like. Keep in mind that the real purpose of the remaining columns is to help physicians and physician leaders interpret the provider data. Here is where several of the design principles that the design group determined earlier come into play.

Comparative data vs. targets

Comparative data are used to compare an individual physician with other physicians, either within the physician's own hospital or as part of a larger normative database. Targets are necessary to consistently interpret data. Providing comparative averages of data with some normative group such as the physicians' department average or the national average is often seen as helpful to many medical staffs. Whether this truly aids in interpretation or is merely a traditional way to look at data is not yet clear. If your medical staff desires these comparisons in addition to targets, there is certainly no harm in including them, other than making the report more crowded. But comparative data are not a substitute for targets.

Number of targets

To create an improvement culture, there should be two target columns for the excellence and acceptable targets, respectively.

CHAPTER 11

Symbolic data interpretation: Using summary rating symbols

Although you can present data in multiple ways, you must present them in a manner that your medical staff will understand. An effective physician performance feedback report does not need to provide a high level of detail to help physicians identify areas of excellence and improvement.

A primary goal in designing feedback reports is to turn data into information and to turn that information into action. Visual symbolic formats provide the best methods for data interpretation. This is typically called a scorecard or summary-rating format, in which a symbol is provided to help the reader quickly interpret the data. Although graphs can also be used to visually display data, the number of indicators that will be needed to evaluate physician competency makes it cumbersome to create a graph for each measure. Consider using a summary-rating symbol as a column on the feedback report to indicate the level of performance for each indicator.

Colors or symbols are most often used to display the performance rating. The goal is to use a scheme that people naturally recognize. For instance, green, yellow, and red are easy: Green means excellent performance; yellow means acceptable; and red means follow-up is needed. Colors are ideal in that they quickly draw the reader's attention first to the interpretation, rather than to the detail of the data. Other examples of symbol schemes are:

- The characters +, 0, and –

- One, three, and five stars

- Up, down, and horizontal arrows

- Smiling, neutral, and frowning faces (pediatric hospitals like these)

One reason graphs are used is to show trends. However, summary-rating symbols can also be used to show trends by having additional columns with the summary-rating symbol displayed from previous rating periods. For example, using the color-scheme approach, the reader can easily see whether the general level of performance has changed over time. Has a red become a yellow or even a green? Has a yellow dropped to a red?

Figure 11.1 shows a feedback report that incorporates the design principles and formatting concepts discussed in this chapter. Figure 11.2 provides an explanation of a summary-rating report over time.

OPPE PROFILES AND PHYSICIAN PERFORMANCE FEEDBACK

Sample Physician Profile Report

Physician Profile Report - Draft

Provider: Brown, Jerry   **ID:** 109   **Category:** Active   **Specialty:** Internal Medicine

Activity

Time Period	ID#	Indicator Title	Volume
1 Yr End 2011 Qtr 4	1	# of Admissions	35
1 Yr End 2011 Qtr 4	2	# of Consultations	86

Patient Care

Time Period	ID#	Indicator Title	Indicator Type	Numerator	Acceptable Value	Excellence Value	Score
1 Yr End 2011 Qtr 4	8	Blood component use not meeting appropriateness criteria including autologous units	Rule	5	3	1	Red

Time Period	ID#	Indicator Title	Indicator Type	Volume	Numerator	Actual	Expected	Index	Acceptable Value	Excellence Value	Score
6 Mo End 2011 Qtr 2	39	Risk adjusted complications index for medical DRGs	Rate	155		0.0	0.1	0.3	1.3	0.9	Green
6 Mo End 2011 Qtr 2	70	Severity adjusted complications index DRG 89	Rate	255		1.5	2.7	0.6	1.3	0.9	Green

Medical Knowledge

Time Period	ID#	Indicator Title	Indicator Type	Volume	Numerator	Results	Acceptable Value	Excellence Value	Score
9 Mo End 2012 Qtr 3	61	% AMI patients prescribed beta blocker at discharge	Rate	104	102	98.1%	80.0%	95.0%	Green
9 Mo End 2012 Qtr 3	65	% HF patients prescribed ACE/ARB at discharge	Rate	109	101	92.7%	85.0%	95.0%	Yellow

Practice Based Learning

Time Period	ID#	Indicator Title	Indicator Type	Volume	Numerator	Results	Acceptable Value	Excellence Value	Score
1 Yr End 2011 Qtr 4	32	% excellent ratings on physician feedback reports	Rate	28	25	89.3%	50.0%	80.0%	Green

Peer Review- Confidential Information

Dept. Chair _____ Date _____

Thursday, December 06, 2012

CHAPTER 11

Sample Physician Profile Report

11.1

Physician Profile Report - Draft

Provider: Brown, Jerry   ID: 109   Category: Active   Specialty: Internal Medicine

Interpersonal & Communication

Time Period	ID#	Indicator Title	Indicator Type	Numerator	Acceptable Value	Excellence Value	Score
1 Yr End 2011 Qtr 4	12	Orders for restraint not in compliance with JCAHO guidelines	Rule	2	2	0	Yellow
1 Yr End 2011 Qtr 4	20	Physician documentation lacking essential elements per regulatory guideline	Rule	3	4	1	Yellow

Professionalism

Time Period	ID#	Indicator Title	Indicator Type	Numerator	Acceptable Value	Excellence Value	Score
1 Yr End 2011 Qtr 4	15	# of validated incidents of nonavailability for ED call/yr	Rule	2	3	0	Yellow
1 Yr End 2011 Qtr 4	16	# of validated incidents of inappropriate physician behavior/yr	Rule	0	2	0	Green

System Based Practice

Time Period	ID#	Indicator Title	Indicator Type	Numerator	Acceptable Value	Excellence Value	Score
1 Yr End 2011 Qtr 4	21	Validated incidents of physician non compliance with Universal Protocol	Rule	2	1	0	Red

Peer Review–Confidential Information   Date _____
Dept. Chair _____

Thursday, December 06, 2012

OPPE PROFILES AND PHYSICIAN PERFORMANCE FEEDBACK

Sample Provider History Report

11.1

Provider History Report

Provider: Brown, Jerry   ID: 109   Category: Active   Specialty: Internal Medicine

ID#	Indicator Title	Indicator Type	6 Mo Ending 2010 Qtr 4	6 Mo Ending 2011 Qtr 2	6 Mo Ending 2011 Qtr 4	6 Mo Ending 2012 Qtr 2	Acceptable Target	Excellence Target
1	# of Admissions	Activity	57	35	121	45		
2	# of Consultations	Activity	208	86	34	68		

Patient Care

ID#	Indicator Title	Indicator Type	6 Mo Ending 2010 Qtr 4	6 Mo Ending 2011 Qtr 2	6 Mo Ending 2011 Qtr 4	6 Mo Ending 2012 Qtr 2	Acceptable Target	Excellence Target
5	# of cases deemed care controversial	Rate	0 Green	0 Green	0 Green	2 Red	3	0
8	Blood component use not meeting appropriateness criteria including autologous units	Rate	0 Green	2 Red	3 Red	5 Red	3	1

ID#	Indicator Title	Indicator Type	6 Mo Ending 2010 Qtr 4	6 Mo Ending 2011 Qtr 2	6 Mo Ending 2011 Qtr 4	6 Mo Ending 2012 Qtr 2	Acceptable Target	Excellence Target
39	Risk adjusted complications index for medical DRGs	Rate	36.8 Red	0.3 Green	0.4 Green	2.0 Red	1.3	0.9
70	Severity adjusted complications index: DRG 89	Rate	1.0 Yellow	1.4 Red	0.7 Green	1.0 Yellow	1.3	0.9

Medical Knowledge

ID#	Indicator Title	Indicator Type	6 Mo Ending 2010 Qtr 4	6 Mo Ending 2011 Qtr 2	6 Mo Ending 2011 Qtr 4	6 Mo Ending 2012 Qtr 2	Acceptable Target	Excellence Target
61	% AMI patients prescribed beta blocker at discharge	Rate	88.2% Yellow	100.0% Green	100.0% Green	98.8% Green	80.0%	95.0%
65	% HF patients prescribed ACE/ARB at discharge	Rate	78.6% Red	77.3% Red	84.4% Red	104.5% Green	85.0%	95.0%

Practice Based Learning

ID#	Indicator Title	Indicator Type	6 Mo Ending 2010 Qtr 4	6 Mo Ending 2011 Qtr 2	6 Mo Ending 2011 Qtr 4	6 Mo Ending 2012 Qtr 2	Acceptable Target	Excellence Target
32	% excellent ratings on physician feedback reports	Rate	100.0% Green	88.2% Green	90.9% Green	94.6% Green	50.0%	80.0%

Peer Review– Confidential Information
Dept. Chair _____ Date _____

Thursday, December 06, 2012

CHAPTER 11

Sample Provider History Report

11.1

Provider History Report

Provider: Brown, Jerry **ID:** 109 **Category:** Active **Specialty:** Internal Medicine

Interpersonal & Communication

ID#	Indicator Title	Indicator Type	6 Mo Ending 2010 Qtr 4	6 Mo Ending 2011 Qtr 2	6 Mo Ending 2011 Qtr 4	6 Mo Ending 2012 Qtr 2	Acceptable Target	Excellence Target
12	Orders for restraint not in compliance with JCAHO guidelines	Rule	0 Green	2 Red	0 Green	0 Green	2	0
20	Physician documentation lacking essential elements per regulatory guideline	Rule	0 Green	2 Yellow	1 Yellow	0 Green	4	1
22	Suspensions for delinquent medical records	Rule	2 Red	0 Green	0 Green	0 Green	3	0

Professionalism

ID#	Indicator Title	Indicator Type	6 Mo Ending 2010 Qtr 4	6 Mo Ending 2011 Qtr 2	6 Mo Ending 2011 Qtr 4	6 Mo Ending 2012 Qtr 2	Acceptable Target	Excellence Target
14	Validated incidents of physician failure to respond with direct communication to nursing requests fo	Rule	0 Green	0 Green	0 Green	1 Yellow	2	0
15	# of validated incidents of nonavailability for ED call-yr	Rule	0 Green	0 Green	2 Red	0 Green	3	0
16	# of validated incidents of inappropriate physician behavior/yr	Rule	1 Yellow	0 Green	0 Green	0 Green	2	0

System Based Practice

ID#	Indicator Title	Indicator Type	6 Mo Ending 2010 Qtr 4	6 Mo Ending 2011 Qtr 2	6 Mo Ending 2011 Qtr 4	6 Mo Ending 2012 Qtr 2	Acceptable Target	Excellence Target
21	Validated incidents of physician non compliance with Universal Protocol	Rule	0 Green	2 Red	0 Green	0 Green	1	0

Peer Review- Confidential Information
Dept. Chair_____ Date_____

Thursday, December 06, 2012

OPPE PROFILES AND PHYSICIAN PERFORMANCE FEEDBACK

11.2 Explanation of Scorecard Format

The sample scorecard format in Figure 11.1 contains the elements described below. The data and the targets are illustrative examples and are not based on actual data or literature.

Activity data: The amount of work in the organization (e.g., admissions, procedures, consults) a physician completes within a given time period.

Performance data: Measures of the results of physician activity either using outcome or process indicators. In this column, the specific indicators should be grouped by physician performance dimension (e.g., technical quality, service quality).

Indicator type: Rule, review, or rate.

Physician volume: The activity level for that particular indicator. For rate indicators, the volume data is the denominator for the rate. For rule indicators, the volume is not applicable (N/A) because the rule is based on individual incidents.

Physician data: The results specific to that physician's performance for that indicator.

Excellence performance target: The threshold or target that separates excellent performance from acceptable performance.

Acceptable performance target: The threshold or target that separates acceptable performance from performance that needs follow-up.

Target source: The information system, committee, or benchmark that is the source of the target selection (e.g., information systems, peer review committee).

Current rating: The color or symbol that indicates the relationship of the provider's data to the targets for that indicator for the current measurement period.

How will the data be understood?

After you have interpreted the data, you will need to understand the data better, particularly if an indicator falls below the acceptable targets. (Ironically, physicians have rarely asked to explore the reliability or accuracy of their own data if the indicators show excellent performance.) For effective feedback, a report needs to be concise, so extensive explanation is not really feasible. Instead, the report needs good support materials and clear information regarding whom to contact to get further information or explanation. The next section will describe the support materials in greater detail.

Prepare and Distribute Competency Data Reports

Once you have defined the principles and designed the format for your physician competency report, you are ready to bring your report to life. Think of it like the story of Pinocchio®, in which the woodcarver Geppetto creates a puppet, but the puppet must learn and experience much more before he can become a real boy.

At this point in the process, you've done a lot of work, but you must take two more steps to make your report "real": develop infrastructure and support materials and pilot-test your design to ensure that it is effective.

Each step is necessary for the long-term success of your report. Organizations often feel pressured to get a competency report out quickly and then pay for it in the long run because of their inability to follow through with a systematic report process. The goal is to develop a report that is not a one-time event, but rather will be provided to physicians every six months.

Keep in mind that the first physician competency report you distribute to your medical staff doesn't have to be perfect or include data on all of the general competencies. I recommend the crawl, walk, run approach to getting started and keeping that momentum moving forward. The key is to have a plan that defines when you can move from crawling to walking and what it will take to move from walking to running.

Develop the Infrastructure and Support Materials

You need three components to support your feedback report process:

- The computer systems to produce the report

- The staff to prepare and distribute the report

- The materials to explain the report

Although support systems vary based on institutional resources, all organizations must secure support from computer systems and staff. When planning your feedback report distribution, identify your capabilities and gaps in each of these areas.

Computer support

Begin to assess your needs for computer support by asking two questions:

- How will you get the data into and out of your current computer systems?

- Will you need additional computer systems or software applications to make this happen?

Many organizations collect enormous amounts of data but struggle to get that data into a common format for inclusion in the competency data report. Others may have data collected on paper that they need to put into some electronic format. To solve these challenges, organizations may have to purchase a sophisticated information system, modify current systems, or simply use common PC software to create a database.

When devising a plan to tackle computer system challenges, work with your IT department. Having an IT representative on your competency report design group will help to shape the feedback report. Don't wait until you've designed your reports to engage your IT team.

Staff support

Even today's sophisticated computer systems can do only so much. You need staff members to prepare and distribute your physician competency report. Although there is clearly a need for support for data collection, for the purposes of this chapter we will focus on the staff support required for assembly and distribution of competency reports.

Staff support for these reports typically comes from two areas:

- Quality department

- Medical staff services department (MSSD)

Who does what varies based on the resources and focus of each department and the culture of the medical staff regarding how each group is perceived. For example, in many organizations, the quality department may be responsible for preparing the report, but the MSSD may distribute it because the MSSD is the recognized source of distribution for most medical staff materials. Therefore, the medical staff may be more comfortable if it receives medical staff–related documents from the MSSD. In some cases, the MSSD may have direct access to the software that produces the report, so it will carry out both functions. Conversely, in some organizations, the quality department may take on the task of collecting data and distributing the reports.

Different methods of distribution will have an impact on the resources needed. Consider the following questions:

- **Will reports be sent electronically?** Most organizations print and distribute the reports manually, which requires staff time to place the reports in envelopes and label them accurately. Sending the reports electronically would reduce the amount of staff time needed to send out the reports.

- **How will physicians receive competency reports?** If you choose not to send the reports electronically, you must decide whether you will mail the reports, deliver them to physician offices, or hand them out at medical staff or department meetings. Remember, it is important to protect the confidentiality of your physician competency data. For example, I don't recommend placing the reports in physicians' mailboxes because others have access to those mailboxes as well.

- **What information will be sent with the competency reports?** Decide which materials to send along with the competency report and which to make available online or at the MSSD. For example, although you could send a glossary with every report, many organizations simply have it available via electronic means or in the MSSD.

When determining how much support you need to distribute your competency reports, consider whether you may need to budget for temporary help for one week every six months to get the reports out without burdening your staff. You may also opt to time the six-month distributions during "slow" periods for the office, which, of course, is all relative.

Support materials

In addition to the report itself, you must provide physicians with additional materials to help them understand the report. The goal of most reports is to be concise and easy to read. Therefore, it is best

OPPE PROFILES AND PHYSICIAN PERFORMANCE FEEDBACK

not to include more explanatory detail than necessary on the actual report. The following four types of support materials are helpful:

- A report cover letter: This is typically from the medical staff president or peer review committee chair (or signed by both). It should be brief and explain the medical staff's ownership of the report, the reason the report is being sent, and the philosophy behind the use of the data.

- An explanation of the report format: This is usually a brief document that accompanies each report and describes the purpose of each column on the report as well as explains how to interpret the colors or symbols used.

- A glossary of terms and indicators: This is a more substantial document that provides the physician with greater detail regarding the indicators and the terms used in the report. For each indicator, the glossary should define the following:

    - Reason for selection

    - Data source

    - Target source

    - How rate measures are calculated

    - Typical factors that could contribute to below-acceptable results

- FAQs: Putting together frequently asked questions (FAQ) is a useful change management strategy. The FAQs should address how the report was created, who selected the measures, how the data should be interpreted, and how the organization will use the data. FAQs are especially helpful when distributing competency reports for the first time and when sharing such reports with new medical staff members. You can use the 10 questions that you used to design your report (p. 159) for your FAQs.

With these materials in hand, you are now ready to distribute your physician competency report. Or are you? How confident are you that your design will be received the way it was intended? Although the simplest short-term strategy is to send out the report and see what happens, adding an extra step of pilot-testing to your report can provide a higher probability of long-term success.

CHAPTER 11

Pilot-Test Your Design

Designing a pilot test need not be a complicated endeavor. It is simply an additional step that provides valuable supplementary information to make final-course adjustments before going forward at full speed. Although you should always be open to feedback regarding improvements in your report, your goal is to actively solicit feedback during the pilot-test phase.

The first step of pilot-testing is to develop a brief work plan. These three questions can guide your work plan:

1. What will you test? Organizations often focus the pilot test only on the accuracy of the data. The pilot test is a great opportunity to look at all of the components, including the following:

    - The acceptability of the indicators

    - The accuracy of the initial data

    - Whether the format is understandable

    - The impact of the cover letter to the staff

    - The usefulness of the glossary

    - The mechanism for distribution

2. Who will be your pilot-test group? The goal of the pilot test is to get a representative sample of feedback to be sure that what you have designed is not biased toward one group. Physicians in various specialties often have different perspectives. Although your design group should be a reasonable representation of physician specialties, the pilot test can give you a broader perspective. Also, because the design group is close to the work product, they may not see flaws that will be apparent to a fresh set of eyes. Here are a few options for selecting a pilot-test group:

    - A single or a few departments

    - Members of a current medical staff committee

- A sample of practitioners from each major specialty

Although it may be tempting to start with a single department because you will need to produce only one type of report, this approach limits both the feedback you receive and the ultimate distribution of the report across the medical staff. Working with three major departments that comprise a significant portion of your medical staff (e.g., medicine, surgery, and OB-GYN) is an option but can be a cumbersome way to get the feedback.

Working with a sample of physicians is generally a more efficient way to get the information you need from your pilot test. This could be done by using an existing multi-specialty group, such as the medical executive committee or the peer review committee, or a specially selected group.

3. How will you get feedback? You can obtain feedback in a number of ways depending on the group you have selected. Think in terms of how a manufacturing company obtains feedback when it designs a new product. Typically, it has the marketing department or firm obtain feedback in a number of ways from potential customers. Here are some of the options for obtaining feedback:

- Sending a written survey

- Meeting one-on-one with individuals

- Discussing at routine committee/department meetings

- Conducting small focus group sessions (comprising six to eight individuals)

Sending out a survey is the simplest method. Figure 11.3 shows a sample survey. The advantage of surveys is that they can provide quantitative and qualitative data from a broad group. The disadvantage is that written surveys lack the richness of discussion provided by the other methods.

One-on-one meetings provide great feedback but can be time-consuming and lack the benefits of dialogue among multiple individuals. Routine department meetings provide the potential for dialogue but can be difficult to control in terms of getting clear feedback with a large group.

11.3 Physician Competency Report Focus Group Questionnaire

Specialty: ❏ Surgical ❏ Medical ❏ OB/GYN ❏ Pediatrics ❏ Emergency ❏ Diagnostic

Instructions: For each statement below, please circle the answer that best describes your personal view concerning the information in the statement.

1. The medical staff should be providing physicians with a routine feedback report.

1	2	3	4	5
Strongly Disagree	Disagree	Neutral	Agree	Strongly Agree

2. The report should include data on physician performance in addition to clinical quality (e.g., service quality, patient safety, resource use, relationships, citizenship).

1	2	3	4	5
Strongly Disagree	Disagree	Neutral	Agree	Strongly Agree

3. Physician competency reports should provide positive feedback to recognize excellence as well as targets for acceptable performance.

1	2	3	4	5
Strongly Disagree	Disagree	Neutral	Agree	Strongly Agree

4. The format of the physician competency report is easy to read.

1	2	3	4	5
Strongly Disagree	Disagree	Neutral	Agree	Strongly Agree

5. The physician competency report data is easy to interpret.

1	2	3	4	5
Strongly Disagree	Disagree	Neutral	Agree	Strongly Agree

6. The explanatory materials were helpful for understanding what each indicator was measuring.

1	2	3	4	5
Strongly Disagree	Disagree	Neutral	Agree	Strongly Agree

7. The indicators selected for the report are reasonable measures of physician performance.

1	2	3	4	5
Strongly Disagree	Disagree	Neutral	Agree	Strongly Agree

8. The indicator targets selected by the medical staff appear appropriate.

1	2	3	4	5
Strongly Disagree	Disagree	Neutral	Agree	Strongly Agree

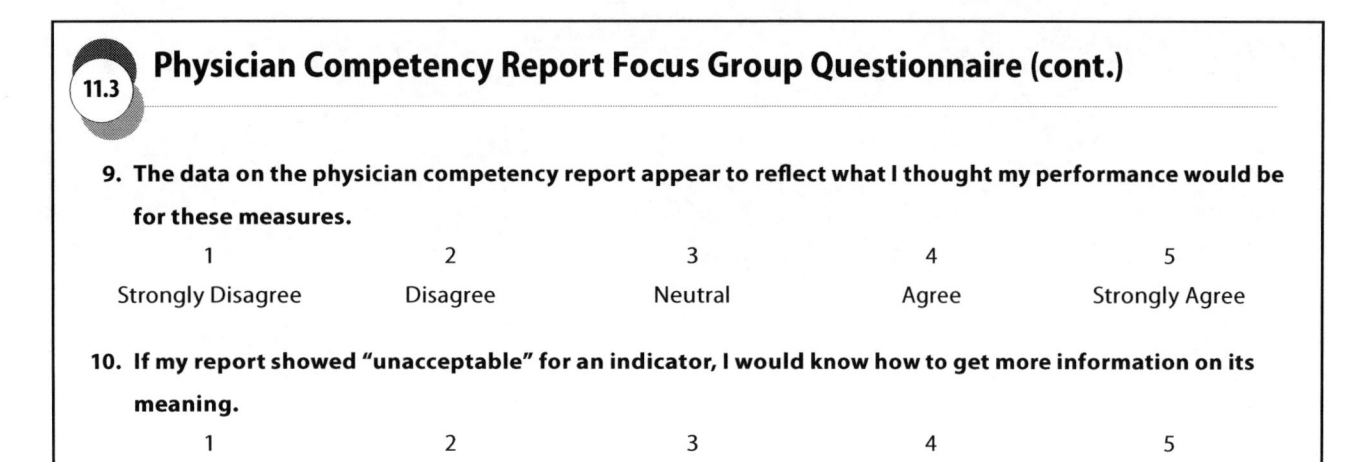

> **11.3 Physician Competency Report Focus Group Questionnaire (cont.)**
>
> 9. **The data on the physician competency report appear to reflect what I thought my performance would be for these measures.**
>
> | 1 | 2 | 3 | 4 | 5 |
> |---|---|---|---|---|
> | Strongly Disagree | Disagree | Neutral | Agree | Strongly Agree |
>
> 10. **If my report showed "unacceptable" for an indicator, I would know how to get more information on its meaning.**
>
> | 1 | 2 | 3 | 4 | 5 |
> |---|---|---|---|---|
> | Strongly Disagree | Disagree | Neutral | Agree | Strongly Agree |

Small focus groups seem to provide the best approach if you can convince physicians to commit the time to attend. You can encourage participation by offering an incentive (e.g., a gift certificate). The focus groups could be composed of physicians of similar specialties or of different specialties. You may need only one group, but often, having two groups at different times of the day (e.g., early morning and early evening) can help to attract physicians with differing practice schedules. Figure 11.4 shows a sample letter inviting physicians to a focus group.

Create a Policy for Physician Competency Reports

Now that you have the information you need to move forward with your feedback report distribution, it is important to create a written policy and procedures. These documents should include all of the decisions your design group has made, as well as reflect everything learned through pilot testing.

11.4 Sample Focus Group Letter Survey

Date:

Name:

Address:

Dear Dr. _____:

Thank you for participating in the focus group for physician competency feedback reports. We appreciate your willingness to share your time, expertise, and input in this valuable process. We will be meeting with you and your peers to facilitate discussion about the report and to seek your feedback regarding its content.

In preparation for that discussion, you will find enclosed your report, which shows your specific data. Please do not share this with others as this is a draft report. You will also find enclosed a glossary that defines each indicator, its source, and why it is deemed an important measure of physician performance.

At the meeting we will be seeking feedback on the following aspects of the report:
Report content: What is being measured?
Report format: How is it presented?
Glossary: Does it provide an adequate explanation?
Distribution cover letter: Does it help physicians understand why they are receiving the report?

We have attached a brief survey for you to complete to help quantify your feedback. Please bring this to your focus group session.

We look forward to meeting with you on (insert date), at _____
_____ (time and place). _____ (meal) will be provided.

Sincerely,

Chief of Staff
Chair, Medical Staff Performance Committee

OPPE PROFILES AND PHYSICIAN PERFORMANCE FEEDBACK

SOLVING THE SOFTWARE DATA INPUT CHALLENGE

In the first edition of this book, we provided a Microsoft® Excel® spreadsheet template in which the hospital staff could list the indicators and targets and the red, yellow, and green interpretation would automatically appear. Unfortunately, the tool required that each profile be manually entered into the spreadsheet. In working with hospitals over the years, I received requests to automate the process. I have worked with the The Greeley Company and HCPro to meet this need by creating a Microsoft Access® database. Discussing all features of the Access database product is beyond the scope of this book. (Visit *www.hcmarketplace.com* to learn more about Physician Profile Reporter. However, one issue worth addressing is the challenge of getting data into an OPPE reporting system from multiple data sources.

Physician competency data comes from many different sources, particularly in light of the data needed to measure physician performance relative to the six general competencies. While some programs may have electronic interfaces with the hospital mainframe system, not all the data for OPPE will be found there. For example, severity-adjusted data and core-measure abstracted data come from separate sources. Many organizations may have manually collected data or peer-review case findings that are captured in a separate software program.

The key question is from how many sources are you currently capturing data? I recommend conducting a complete inventory of all your current physician-specific indicators with the data source outlined. Doing so will enable the quality department to get a handle on collecting, analyzing, and disseminating data.

So what is the solution to the multiple data source challenge? Since large data acquisition systems are not designed to easily accept imported data without a programmed electronic interface, the solution is to require the reporting software program to accept data from multiple sources that may not have a direct interface. When the physician profile reporter was developed with this feature via importing data in an Excel format, few profile software systems had this capability. Today, this is becoming more common and there are several vendors that offer the capability of receiving data for a variety of sources at varying cost levels. It is important to ask a prospective software vendor whether their system has this capability.

12 External Peer Review in a Physician Improvement Culture

There are two processes that medical staffs typically use to obtain physician reviewers for case review: internal peer review (IPR) and external peer review (EPR). Although these are often seen as separate silos of the peer review function, I think they are best viewed as tools that use different resources to acquire fair, efficient, and useful information to evaluate and improve physician performance. To do both of these functions well, organizations need solid IPR systems and clear policies for obtaining and using EPR evaluations. Chapter 2 discussed the IPR process. This chapter will focus on EPR.

EPR Uses

EPR is typically thought of as the review of a medical record for individual cases in which concerns have been raised regarding the quality or appropriateness of care. This can be based on adverse outcomes, the appropriateness of procedures or treatments, or the use of resources. For the purposes of this book, we will focus primarily on the use of EPR for case reviews, but we thought it important to mention the broader uses as well. They are:

- Focused professional practice review (FPPE) of randomly selected cases to determine frequency of outcomes or patterns of care

- Prior to exercising privileges, such as in the evaluation of a credential file for initial appointment

- Direct observation of practitioner technique, skill, or knowledge

- Monitoring following the implementation of a quality improvement plan for a physician or department

The EPR Policy

EPR should be driven by a clear medical staff policy. Legal counsel should review any policy related to implementation of an outside review. Once the decision is made to consider external peer review, follow to the letter the medical staff bylaws, peer review policy, and any other related medical staff policies. A good EPR policy should address the following six questions:

- What circumstances typically require EPR?
- Who determines when EPR is needed?
- Who will select the reviewer?
- How will the cases be selected?
- Who will review the EPR report findings?
- How will the results be used?

Using this as a framework, we will discuss how your policy can address each of these questions.

What Circumstances Typically Require EPR?

The hospital peer review policy must make it clear when EPR will be used. Typically, EPR is recommended under the following circumstances:

- Lack of internal expertise
- Ambiguity
- Credibility
- Legal concerns
- Benchmarking
- Lack of internal resources

Let's explore each of these reasons in more depth.

EXTERNAL PEER REVIEW IN A PHYSICIAN IMPROVEMENT CULTURE

Lack of internal expertise

EPR can be viewed as a supplement to your stable of internal reviewers. This can be due to two reasons. The first is because of a recognized, ongoing need. For example, if there is only one neurosurgeon on your medical staff, you will always need external review for specialty-specific issues related to that surgeon. The second reason is because of a more time-limited need. This is due to the introduction of new technology or a new procedure at your hospital when no one on the medical staff has that privilege elsewhere (e.g., robotic prostatectomy). Eventually, if more than one member of your staff uses that technology or privilege, you will be able to conduct the review internally.

Ambiguity

There are times of honest disagreement in case review that result in vague or conflicting recommendations from internal reviewers or medical staff committees. Obtaining the view of external experts can often settle these issues.

Credibility

EPR can be useful to validate the effectiveness of your internal review process. This is most often due to concerns about conflict of interest when you determine that the physicians with the expertise you need for the case have a conflict (the methods of determining conflict were discussed in Chapter 2). It can also be due to the committee's discomfort with rendering a judgment that will not be well received without external backup. But EPR can also be useful if your peer review process in general does not appear to find issues with physician care very often and the overall credibility of your peer review committee comes into question.

Legal concerns

When issues of physician competence may be addressed in a legal or due process action, EPR can provide the organization with information that can prevent it from adopting the wrong strategy or making the wrong decision. This can include cases that might result in patient litigation or cases that relate to the medical staff corrective action and fair hearing process. In the latter case, the external expert may also be involved as an expert witness for a fair hearing.

Benchmarking

An organization might need benchmarking because it lacks expertise or there is ambiguity. There are times when an organization is concerned about the care provided by its physicians relative to best practices and wishes to better define its expectations. In these instances, the external review is the driving source for improvement and future quality monitoring to determine whether improvement has been achieved.

Lack of internal resources

There are times when an organization wishes to perform a larger study involving many patient records. Even though the medical staff has the internal expertise that is without conflict, there might not be an internal reviewer who has the time. Using external reviewers can expedite the process.

Who Determines When EPR Is Needed?

Typically, recommendations for EPR arise from peer review committees that are faced with issues they can't resolve for the reasons discussed above or from medical staff and hospital leaders dealing with potential legal or credibility issues. The board should also have the right to decide whether it needs EPR to answer concerns or protect itself legally even if the medical staff believes it can, or has, conducted a fair review. Although a physician may ask that the committee or leadership request EPR for his or her case, I strongly recommend that your policy not allow for the involved physician to have the right to demand EPR. It is the organization's decision whether it can perform peer review fairly. That said, wise organizations should consider the physician's concerns in making their decision, particularly when dealing with potentially litigious physicians.

Because EPR will often require the use of extra financial resources, the hospital or medical staff leadership should approve the need for EPR. This approval may go through the medical executive committee (MEC) or via a mutual agreement between the medical staff president and an administrative leader, often the vice president for medical affairs or the chief medical officer, if the organization has one. Unless the review is a routine review due to lack of internal expertise, the hospital's legal counsel should clearly identify and support the precipitating reason for the EPR. For example, was the review initiated because of concern that a potential patient-care problem might exist? Was it initiated after an investigation designed to determine whether sanctions are necessary? Was it initiated because support was needed for sanctions already rendered? Appropriately answering these questions can make all the difference between an orderly, collegial solution and an adversarial fair hearing. No outside evaluation should be initiated without involving legal counsel experienced in healthcare law.

One issue sometimes raised is whether an EPR requested by a medical staff peer review committee should be made available to risk management for claims evaluation and whether an EPR requested by risk management should be available to the peer review committee to guide its review. While it would

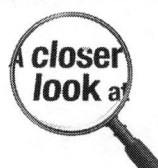

EXTERNAL PEER REVIEW IN A PHYSICIAN IMPROVEMENT CULTURE

A closer look at: How to Select Appropriate External Peer Reviewers

People select their physicians in two ways: prospectively before they are sick or more urgently when a sudden illness occurs. However, very few individuals select all the specialists they might need in case they get sick. This is typically done by choosing a primary care provider who can then guide them in the selection of the right specialist when they need one.

Selecting an external reviewer is similar to selecting your physician. It is wise to have potential external peer reviewers in mind because the need for them can arise without warning. This is typically done by identifying an organization, either another hospital or an external peer review (EPR) company that can meet your external review needs for whatever types of cases that arise.

What are the characteristics of a good external review organization? The following list may be helpful:

- Credibility: A good track record of EPR experience and use of currently active, board-certified, clinical consultants in all specialties.

- Objectivity: The ability to ensure that the physician reviewer has no knowledge of or connection to the physician being reviewed. This is typically achieved by using reviewers from other geographic areas. (Note: External peer reviewers do not need to be privileged by the facilities that use their services.)

- Professional report: A description of the review methods, record selection mechanism, case-specific findings, and conclusions or recommendations when requested.

- Timeliness: Defined typical turnaround time frames that meet your needs and the ability to expedite reports when needed.

- Ease of interpretation: The rating system should differentiate between definitive findings and clinical areas in which appropriate treatment is still being debated, and the language should be as specific as possible. Equivocal language that only implies problems leaves the medical executive committee (MEC) with a dilemma. (Note: Although some hospitals request that the external peer reviewers include recommendations in the report, do so only after consulting your attorney. It may be more appropriate for an MEC to arrive at its own conclusions after the report is completed because it must make the final recommendation anyway.)

- Support: Assistance with case selection decisions, willingness to participate in conference calls to clarify the report, and the ability to defend and support findings if a subsequent fair hearing or litigation ensues, including testifying.

- Confidentiality: The ability to commit to absolute confidentiality and strict nondisclosure. Provisions pertaining to confidentiality should be discussed in advance and included in the contract language.

seem that an organization would like to share the information given the expense that may be involved to obtain it, the issue has potential legal repercussions related to peer review protection from discovery and loss of attorney-client privilege for risk management. A good EPR policy should at least address the issue based on advice from legal counsel.

Who Will Select the Reviewer?

Typically, the body with authority to determine whether a review is necessary also selects the reviewer. This is important because there needs to be up-front buy-in regarding the credibility of the reviewer. Although the MEC or quality committee may delegate the preliminary selection of the reviewer to an administrator, the choice should be brought back to that group, or at least to the chair, for final approval. The shaded box on p. 187 discusses the criteria for selecting a reviewer or a review organization.

Should the reviewer be required to meet the approval of the physician being reviewed? I recommend this should not be required by your policy. It is important to be sure to match the reviewer to the experience of the physician being reviewed. It is also best practice to make a good effort to engage the physician in the selection process if possible to increase the likelihood of acceptance of the findings. However, reviewer selection should not be held hostage by a recalcitrant physician.

How Will the Cases Be Selected?

If the need for EPR is to make determinations for specific cases, case selection is not an issue. However, if the need is to obtain a more in-depth understanding of a physician's practice (e.g., FPPE), then case selection is critical to interpreting and using the findings. A good peer review policy does not need to have a detailed description of case selection methods. Rather, it should acknowledge the types of approaches that may be used (e.g., single cases, 100% review, random sampling) and who will determine the selection method appropriate for the question at hand. The latter should be done using the same procedure used for reviewer selection. A good EPR organization should be able to provide you with some assistance with case selection. Below are some practical tips for case selection for FPPE.

Remember that old laxative commercial where the person ponders how many prunes will do the job? Are three enough? Are five too many? When The Joint Commission created the new term—focused professional practice evaluation—in 2007, it did not provide clear answers about how many cases one should select.

EXTERNAL PEER REVIEW IN A PHYSICIAN IMPROVEMENT CULTURE

Given the complicated nature of FPPE, medical staffs should probably be flexible when determining how to approach it. But flexibility can lead to an inadequate evaluation or unnecessary time and expense.

Before you begin selecting records for review, the first step is to ask yourself the following four questions:

- What am I measuring?
- What are my goals?
- How will I interpret the data?
- What are my resources?

Although most organizations want to start by determining sample method and size, these questions should determine which records you choose to review. Let's discuss each question a bit further.

What am I measuring?

Unless you define what you are measuring, you might not get the right answer. For example, some reviews are concerned with a particular outcome. Others focus on the use of particular practice or compliance with a policy.

Then there is the more complex issue of whether a physician used good judgment.

What are my goals?

Different goals require different approaches. For example, are you trying to determine whether something is occurring or why it is occurring? The answer would affect the level of detail and expertise needed to conduct a focused review. Are you seeking to understand current competency or improved performance? The answer would affect how far into the past, or the future, you need to go.

How will I interpret the data?

Unless you decide how you will interpret data up front, you might introduce bias into the focused review process.

For example, are you trying to establish statistical significance or a reasonable understanding? The former is more expensive and might not be achievable. Yet if you don't decide that in advance, physicians will often refute the findings. The other factor is the comparison group. Are you comparing the physician to others, to a best practice, or to previous performance?

What are my resources?

A reasonable FPPE design that you can afford is better than an ideal design that you can't. Considering the effect of cost on your goals might not sound very scientific, but it is appropriate because it allows you to revisit your goals to see whether there is an alternative approach that gets you to the answer you need.

Just like using the prunes, performing FPPE usually isn't a pleasant task. Hopefully, these tips will help you get the job done but without overdoing it.

Who Will Review the EPR Report Findings?

Prior to contemplating a corrective action, an EPR report should not be treated any differently than an internal review. The results should be reported to the group that made the initial recommendation—the same group that would be considering the results of an internal review. This is typically the medical staff quality committee or department chair. A good EPR policy also designates a time frame for reviewing the report. This makes the process fairer for the individual under review. Typically, reports should be reviewed within 30 days of receipt or at the next regularly scheduled committee meeting.

An important legal concept to keep in mind is that, after receiving an EPR report, you should not have a specialty department vote on its acceptance. Doing so raises the specter of anticompetitive intent and can provide credibility to an antitrust lawsuit. EPR results should be accepted and acted on by a medical staff credentials or peer review committee or by the MEC, per hospital policy.

Unlike an internal review, in which the committee can query the physician about concerns before coming to a conclusion, an external reviewer must base his or her findings only on medical documentation and image studies provided by the organization. Therefore, if the report identifies any concerns or improvement opportunities, the physician under review should be given an opportunity to review the report and respond in a defined time frame. However, as this is prior to any corrective action process, the physician should not be allowed to have personal legal counsel involved at this stage.

If a corrective action process is being contemplated, the report may go directly to the MEC or its designee. The physician under review and members of any hearing panel (if there is the potential for an adverse action) must have the opportunity to review the results of the evaluation with the individual who conducted the review. They also should be allowed to question the methodology, the outside consultant's qualifications, and the findings in the consultant's report. That is why, if possible, it is best to involve the physician in the reviewer selection process up front.

How Will the Results Be Used?

A good EPR policy should provide guidance on how the results will be interpreted and define the next steps if the results are adverse prior to obtaining an external review. Although a committee should not be constrained regarding its recommendation for improvement or corrective action, it is often helpful to decide whether the findings of the reviewer will be considered definitive. This can be done on a case-by-case basis based on the nature of the review, the expertise of the reviewer, and the issues under review. For example, if the external review is requested merely due to lack of expertise and the reviewer has good credentials, the committee has no real reason to question the findings. On the other hand, if it is a controversial issue, the committee might wish to reserve judgment until reviewing the report to understand the reviewer's rationale for his or her findings.

When considering a recommendation for improvement or action, the medical staff leadership and the MEC should consider the results of the external review along with what they already know about the physician being reviewed. This includes the willingness of the physician to address improvement opportunities. An EPR should not be the only criterion used to take action against a medical staff member.

Beyond Case-Based EPR: Physician Assessment Programs

There may be times when you might want more in-depth scrutiny of a physician's capabilities, strengths, and weaknesses, or when you might wish to provide educational programs to upgrade knowledge and skills. In those instances, an external physician assessment program can be used in place of, or to augment, the peer review process. Such programs can be very expensive, but they could be well worth the cost in certain situations.

Typically, physician assessment programs are more thorough and look at numerous patients when reviewing a physician's abilities. Such programs might include "standardized patient" encounters, in which the physicians are observed as they interview and examine individuals trained to act like patients; written tests; and clinical interviews in the physician's specialty. For more information on a physician assessment program, contact your state medical society.

13. Reporting Peer Review: What Does the Board Need to Know?

In the past, boards of healthcare organizations primarily focused on financial performance, programmatic growth, and capital expansion. Reporting and discussing quality were a relatively small proportion of the meeting time and physician quality an evener smaller proportion of that discussion. The common joke was, just before the chief of staff was about to give the medical staff quality report, typically scheduled at the end of the meeting, the board chair would mention that he or she was running late and could the chief of staff please be brief. Alternatively, the board chair would ask for the medical staff quality report and the chief of staff would simply respond, "Quality is fine and there are no issues." Underlying the brevity of either of these two scenarios is the assumption of most board members that they were not knowledgeable enough to understand healthcare quality and it would be best to leave quality matters in the hands of healthcare professionals.

Contemporary Board Accountabilities for Hospital Quality

What are today's boards hearing about their role? No matter which conference you attend or healthcare magazine you read, there are two major themes:

1. The board is accountable for quality of care, not just finance

2. The board needs to be more engaged in quality initiatives

Of course, board members are not expected to become quality experts and take over the management of quality any more than they would take over the financial management of the organization. The board still needs to delegate these responsibilities as it has in the past. What is new is that the board is being asked to better understand what it is delegating and to actively hold accountable the leaders responsible for the organization's quality performance, just as it has a reasonable understanding of healthcare finance and holds the CEO and chief financial officer accountable for financial performance. Delegation without understanding can lead to lack of accountability and delegation without accountability is abdication of responsibility.

CHAPTER 13

The obvious question is, "To whom should the board delegate the accountability for quality?" In the vast majority of industries, the answer would be simple: management is responsible for all aspects of quality. However, in healthcare organizations, the Centers for Medicare & Medicaid Services' regulations separate performance evaluation of hospital systems and personnel, which is the responsibility of management, from performance evaluation of licensed independent practitioners, which is the responsibility of the medical staff. Even outside of regulatory-driven settings, most organizations feel that physicians are in the best position to evaluate other physicians. While physicians can and should assist the hospital to improve patient care systems and the hospital needs to provide the resources to help the medical staff address physician performance, the evaluation and improvement of individual and aggregate physician performance is the job the board needs the medical staff to address.

The best goal for the medical staff is to partner with the board in the measurement and improvement of physician quality. Unless, of course, your goal is to be sure the board doesn't care or understand what is going on so it will not get into your business. The problem with that approach is that when something significant does occur, it will be harder to gain the board's support.

What Keeps the Board Awake at Night?

The quote from Stephen Covey, "To be understood, first seek to understand" is a good starting place for the medical staff to fulfill the job delegated to it by the board. To gain an understanding of the board's needs, one question that is useful to ask the board (or any group or individual with oversight responsibilities) is "What keeps you awake at night?" In other words, what drives the board's concerns regarding practitioner competency?

There are two common concerns from boards regarding the insomnia question relative to quality:

1. Are we adequately protecting our community (i.e., preventing patient harm)?

2. Are we adequately protecting our organization (i.e., preventing corporate negligence)?

The first concern is one that is familiar to most physicians. That is why we have credentialing and privileging, to be sure physicians are competent to provide patient care. That is why we have peer review, to continue to evaluate competency and help physicians improve to prevent future patient harm. That is why we have bylaws that define the process needed to remove a physician's membership or privileges if continuing to practice would present a danger to patients. If you are doing these functions effectively, and the board is aware of it, it can sleep better.

The second concern is somewhat less familiar. As mentioned in Chapter 3, the issue moves from whether the practitioner was competent to whether the organization was competent. Negligent credentialing is letting someone do something without the appropriate training and experience. Negligent peer review is the organization not knowing what it should do about a physician's performance, not addressing identified issues, and inadequate processes for either. The consequence of corporate negligence is the plaintiff's ability to seek far greater damages than allowed for individual negligence. These damages can potentially have a great impact on the organization's financial standing for which the board is ultimately responsible.

Filling in the Knowledge Gap: Helping Boards Understand Physician Competency Measurement

Understanding the board's concerns helps to define the strategy to address it. Clearly, to meet its responsibilities for medical staff quality, the board needs more than just quality data. To have confidence in the data, the board needs a reasonable understanding of how the data was produced. It also needs to know how the data is evaluated and what is done with the results. This is no different than the expectation that financial data should be accompanied by an explanation of the accounting practices used and any actions taken to address financial shortfalls. So what systems are involved in producing and evaluating physician performance data?

There are four main systems that should be explained to the board:

1. The case review process

2. The data systems for obtaining aggregate and practitioner-level data

3. The ongoing professional practice evaluation (OPPE) process

4. The procedure for performing focused professional practice evaluation (FPPE) for OPPE concerns

The simplest—but probably least effective—way to educate board members is to just give it a bunch of polices to read. Effective board education requires some effort to distill the important information into a digestible form. The methods may vary based on the board culture and existing board educational approaches, but here are some best practices:

CHAPTER 13

- Create a board-specific peer review overview packet for new members

- Hold a question-and-answer session to walk them through the peer review program

- Conduct an annual overview presentation

- Allow individual board members to attend and observe a peer review committee meeting as a planned invited guest

This last practice may be viewed as controversial and should only be considered if the board members have clear understanding of the confidential nature of the discussion, the organization's culture promotes transparency, and the medical staff has put in place an effective peer review program. That said, if the medical staff is doing peer review well, nothing helps to gain board credibility more than allowing individual members to observe the process.

One question that is often asked is whether the whole board needs to be educated or just a board subcommittee? The common reason for creating a subcommittee is to allow for in-depth discussion that will save time at the full board meeting. Therefore, one would expect the subcommittee to have a more in-depth understanding of the peer review systems. However, it is recommended that you don't restrict board education to the subcommittee members. Each board member needs some form of education, although it can be briefer than that provided to the subcommittee. Otherwise, when significant issues arise, there may be misunderstandings from the uneducated members regarding the decisions or recommendations of the subcommittee.

What Data Should the Board Get?

While explaining the processes underlying peer review helps to gain board credibility and perhaps grant it a few more hours of sleep, the real proof that peer review is working is based on the saying of W. Edwards Deming, "In God we trust, all others must bring data." The often-asked question is, "What data and how much?"

Although the board is ultimately responsible for physician quality, as with financial oversight, the level of data detail presented should decrease as the level of authority increases. For example, financial data is typically presented to the board in summary ratios that can quickly show whether the financial systems are working properly and if there is a need for action or alarm.

REPORTING PEER REVIEW: WHAT DOES THE BOARD NEED TO KNOW?

Unfortunately, physician performance data does not have the well-established metrics available for financial data reporting. In this new era of quality data, as an industry, we are still making our way through uncharted waters. This point was made to me 10 years ago when I was meeting with a hospital-board quality subcommittee presenting a relative abundance of data, assuming it would help the members understand quality better. The chair asked whether it was possible to boil the data down to a few metrics that the board could track, following the principle of noted architect Ludwig Mies van der Rohe, "Less is more." This led to the following principles that can help guide the development of an effective board report:

- Define mutually agreed-upon measures: It is not uncommon to assume the board doesn't know much about quality data and your job is to decide what data they need. Having an open dialogue with the board (typically the subcommittee) about what it would like to receive is a great way to increase the likelihood that it will better understand what it receives. This conversation should include both the currently available measures as well as how the data might be consolidated in a more aggregate or compact manner.

- Use a consistent format: With data presentation, consistency is king. If you see someone you meet in a work setting, like a hospital, and meet him or her again in a recreational setting, like a soccer game, you may not recognize the person because he or she is wearing different clothes. The same is true for data. Clothing data in different formats makes it harder each time to recognize the data's meaning.

- Present data in an easily interpreted layout: Most organizations are using formats like colored scorecards or symbols that allow easy visual interpretation results. This should include information for the current reporting period and for data trends. The latter is often shown as a symbol, such as arrows up or down to indicate positive or negative trends. Discuss with the board how much detail-level data is really needed so the layout can be reasonably compact and the reader is not overwhelmed by too many columns of figures.

- Provide detail only if needed for action: Too often, detail-level data is presented on every item just in case some might ask. At a board level, detail is only needed if the board is being requested to take some action other than approving the data. If a board member asks about something that is not an action item on the agenda, the issue can be deferred and the supporting data can be provided at the next meeting.

CHAPTER 13

Based on these principles, the board should receive two types of data to understand the effectiveness of peer review:

1. Case review data

2. OPPE/FPPE data

Case review data

To assure the board that case review is working as designed in the policies and procedures, the board should routinely be provided aggregate data on both the efficiency and effectiveness of the case review. However, the board should not receive information regarding the individual physician case review findings. At this point, the board only needs to know that the case review system results in improvements in patient care. Until there is a recommendation related to a specific physician membership or privileges, the board does not need to know the identity of the individuals. Providing the identity on individual cases can lead to premature involvement by the board, or by individual board members—particularly physician members—in the peer review process and may negatively affect efforts to create a performance improvement–focused culture.

For efficiency, provide data on the timeliness of the case review process and how well the case screening system identified cases and eliminated unnecessary physician reviews. For effectiveness, provide aggregate data on the case review decisions and the types of improvement opportunities identified. Figure 13.1 describes an approach The Greeley Company uses that can help you provide the board with this data.

OPPE and FPPE data

For OPPE and FPPE data, like case review, the board routinely needs aggregate data to know whether the OPPE and FPPE system is working and what types of improvement opportunities are being identified regarding individual physician competency. Again, the board does not need to know the identity of the practitioner at this stage unless the improvement effort fails.

Here are the types of data that can fulfill these needs:

- Number of physician outliers for each indicator on OPPE reports

- Number and types of follow-up conclusions following department chair evaluation

REPORTING PEER REVIEW: WHAT DOES THE BOARD NEED TO KNOW?

13.1 How Effective and Efficient Is Your Case Review Program?

Often, medical staffs judge the usefulness of case review by the quantity of cases reviewed rather than by the number of opportunities to improve physician care. Yet physicians and quality support staff members are often left with the feeling that either the right cases aren't being identified for the peer reviewers or the peer review committees aren't willing to make the right call. The Greeley Company's experience in assessing more than 100 hospital peer review programs over the past four years has provided an opportunity to benchmark the results of case review. In the chart below are six data elements that help define the effectiveness and efficiency of the case review process.

Medical staffs can use these six data elements to calculate the five indicators of case review benchmarking further described in the chart on p.200. Although an in-depth discussion of these measures is beyond the scope of this book, we provide them to you along with suggested benchmarks as a means of evaluating your case review process and tracking and reporting this data to your medical executive committee and governing board. The downloadable materials accompanying this book includes a spreadsheet, "PED Data Calculation," that will allow you to enter your data and automatically calculate your results.

The following data elements should be collected for the same time period:

Data element	Description
Number of hospital discharges/year	If less than one year's worth of data is available, provide the approximate number of discharges for that time period.
Number of cases identified for potential physician review through screening or referrals	Number of discharges during time period that were identified by either routine screening indicators or audits to find cases for peer review or referrals (e.g., from case managers, risk management occurrence reports, physicians,) to peer review for consideration for physician review. Do not include cases simply being abstracted for creating rate or rule measures (e.g., core measures, documentation audits).
Number of cases per year sent for physician review	Number of cases sent to a physician reviewer for detailed chart review to make an initial determination whether physician care was appropriate.
Number of cases with final rating other than clinical care appropriate (excluding cases with documentation issues only)	Number of cases that have a final finding other than care appropriate or standard of care met, excluding cases with only documentation deficiencies.
Number of physician review cases with final decision within three months of initial case screen/referral	Time span from date case first identified for review (via screens or when referral is received) to date committee makes a determination on physician care. Time frame required to complete any follow-up action with the physician after the committee final decision is not included.
Number of improvement actions taken for cases with final rating other than clinical care appropriate	Total number of actions taken based on cases reviewed and discussed by committee. Examples of types of actions include: educational letter only; meeting with department chair/physician leader; performance data monitoring; additional continuing medical education; proctoring; required consultation; recommendation for restriction of membership or privileges.

13.1 How Effective and Efficient Is Your Case Review Program? (cont.)

Greeley Case Review Effectiveness Indicators

The following indicators should be calculated using the data elements above:

Note: Interpretation: 2=Excellent
                    1=Acceptable, with opportunity to improve
                    0=Needs significant improvement

Indicator	Description	Interpretation
Case identification effectiveness rate	Numerator: Number of cases identified by screening or referrals x 1,000 Denominator: Number of discharges	2>50 1=25–50 0<25
Percent screening effectiveness	Numerator: Number of cases sent to physician for review Denominator: Number of cases identified by screening or referrals	2<50% 1=50–75% 0>75%
Percent review process efficiency	Numerator: Number of cases with final decision within three months of reviewer assignment Denominator: Number of cases sent to physician for review	2>90% 1=75–90% 0<75%
Review system effectiveness rate	Numerator: Number of cases rated care less than appropriate x 1,000 Denominator: Number of discharges	2>5 1=2–5 0<2
Percent improvement actions	Numerator: Number of cases with improvement actions taken Denominator: Number of cases rated care less than appropriate	2>90% 1=50–90% 0<50%

REPORTING PEER REVIEW: WHAT DOES THE BOARD NEED TO KNOW?

- No action warranted

- Informal discussions

- Number and types of FPPE plans initiated

• Number of FPPEs in progress

• Number of FPPEs completed

For the FPPEs initiated, you may also wish to provide the board with the FPPE plan, like the one discussed in Chapter 10. For completed FPPEs, the board should also be provided with the results relative to the improvement goals of the FPPE plan. Again, in both instances, the physician identity does not need to be shared as long as there is no recommendation affecting membership or privileges to the medical executive committee or the board.

Reporting overall medical staff performance

In addition to the above data on individual physician competency, the board also needs to know the level of performance of the medical staff as a whole for physician-relevant indicators (e.g., the compliance compared to national benchmarks for core measures or mortality rates). The reason for the last item is that it tells the board as to whether the medical staff leadership is meeting its responsibilities to meet board goals and priorities for physician-driven indicators. This should include both indicators on the OPPE reports and data for physician-driven measures whether or not the attribution is accurate at the individual physician level.

In creating such a report, most organizations use a scorecard format with targets for excellence and acceptable performance. Figure 13.2 provides a sample report to give to the board. Although this data may be reported by the hospital quality staff as part of a hospital scorecard, having the physician measures in a medical staff–specific scorecard helps the board to know who is accountable (e.g., medical staff or management) for which measures. It also allows the medical staff report to be organized by core competency and contain internal measures, such as rule measures that would otherwise not appear on the hospital report.

Finally, if any of the indicators on the overall medical staff report indicate an outlier status or a negative trend, the report should include a description of the steps being taken to either identify or correct the cause. To maintain credibility with the board, by the time data is presented, you should always be able to demonstrate that you are not waiting for the board to figure it out.

13.2 Sample Board Reports

Case Review Process Indicators	Results*		Targets	
Indicator	Current 6 months	Previous 6 months	Excellent	Follow-up
Case Identification Effectiveness Rate	75.0	70.0	> 50	<25
% Screening Effectiveness	43%	46%	< 50%	>75%
% Review Process Efficiency (3 months)	70%	80%	> 90%	>75%
Review System Effectiveness Rate	4.4	5.4	> 5.0	<2.0
% Improvement Actions	95%	85%	>90%	<50%
% Documentation Issue Identification	15%	10%	>20%	<5%
% Pt. Safety/PI Issue Identification	8%	2%	>10%	<2.5%

* Highlight results with green, yellow, or red based on targets set. Green = excellent Yellow = acceptable Red = follow-up

OPPE Process

OPPE Indicator Process	Current 6 Months #	%	Previous 6 Months #	%
# Physicians receiving OPPE reports	200		200	
Physicians with indicators in follow-up category	10	5%	15	7.5%
Physicians with department chair follow up with 30 days	8	80%	10	66%
Follow-up findings				
Data error	3	30%	5	33%
Improvement discussion	5	50%	8	54%
FPPE required	2	20%	2	14%

Current FPPEs	Start Date	Projected Completion Date
Core measure compliance (SCIP)	1/13	6/13
Restraint documentation	2/13	4/13
OB complications	7/13	12/13
Chemotherapy protocol use	7/13	9/13

Indicator	Indicator Type	Results	Excellence Target	Acceptable Target	Current score	Previous score
Patient care						
Risk adj. mortality index: All DRGs	Rate	0.95	<0.9	<1.5	Green	Green
Risk adj. complication index	Rate	0.88	<0.9	<1.5	Green	Green
Medical knowledge						
% compliance with core measures	Rate	0.98	<98%	>90%	Green	Yellow
Interpersonal and communication skills						
H&P/OP report not dictated w/in 24 hrs	Rule	4	0	<3	Red	Yellow
Patient satisfaction with MD percentile	Rate	0.65	>75%	>50%	Yellow	Yellow
Systems-based practice						
Severity-adjusted LOS	Rate	0.9	<0.9	<1.5	Green	Green
Delayed starts in OR/procedure area	Rule	1	<4	<8	Green	Green
Professionalism						
Physician behavior incidents	Review	1	0	<3	Yellow	Green
Medical records suspensions	Rule	2	0	<3	Yellow	Green

14: Running an Effective Peer Review Committee Meeting

Physician leaders are often expected to perform responsibilities for which they have received no training. Some of those responsibilities are technical, like evaluating privileges. But more general leadership responsibilities that require training can have a major impact on the medical staff if not performed well. One of those critical responsibilities is running a committee meeting.

The Greeley Company is often asked to speak at medical staff retreats on how to run an effective committee meeting. In one instance, I received a request from the incoming medical staff president who had observed that many of the committee meetings were not well run. As a good leader, he realized that most of the incoming leaders, either as department chairs or specific committee chairs, had not been provided with any formal or informal guidance on how to ensure they were putting their voluntary time to its best use.

Except for the complimentary donuts, physicians often dislike medical staff meetings because they are usually volunteering their time and are losing either time at their practice or at home. While they are willing to perform this sacrifice if they feel it has value, unfortunately, they often find these meetings are unproductive. Here are some common reasons why:

- Late starts so meetings run late

- Poor preparation so discussions are not well guided or members don't have adequate information to make a decision

- Controversial topics take over the agenda so planned business doesn't get done

- Discussion monopolized by a few individuals who repeat the same points

- Grandstanding or axe grinding because a physician is not on the committee that deals with the issue at hand and this is the only venue he or she has to vent

CHAPTER 14

- Ceremonial dog and pony shows from quality staff to "educate" physicians or to get credit for their work

- Desire for unanimous approval of everything so expression of minority views disproportionately prolong discussions and prevent decisions

With physician participation in medical staff affairs declining, if left unaddressed, these issues can lead to further loss of willing participants.

Most organizations underestimate the true cost of a medical staff meeting because the cost is hidden. Most importantly, is the opportunity cost absorbed by the physicians in terms of lost income that is created by taking them out of their practices to attend meetings. This cost is far beyond the cost of any stipends physicians might be paid as discussed in Chapter 1. The opportunity cost could be well over $10,000 for a one-hour meeting involving 10 physicians. The other cost to consider is the support staff cost to prepare and attend the meeting. The question to ask yourself is "Are you getting your money's worth?" For most medical staffs, the answer is "No."

So what can you do about it? Actually, quite a lot once you recognize that meeting management is a learned skill rather than an inherent competency. It has a number of techniques that are fairly well understood in the corporate world. While it is true that some people will naturally run a meeting better than others, everyone can do it better with some training. Although physician leaders tend to resist "management" training, if they are willing to accept the concept that being generally smart does not eliminate the need for training on specific skills, they can greatly help their medical staff.

Elements of an Effective Meeting

The aim of a good meeting is to make decisions, not pander to emotional expression, endless processing, or social gathering. So what are the specific things that you can learn to run an effective peer review committee meeting? I have found at least four key elements that apply to many types of meetings but are particularly useful for peer review committees:

- Meeting preparation: Making sure the agenda is well planned and decision support materials are available and clear

- Agenda management: Sticking with the agenda to ensure important issues get their due

RUNNING AN EFFECTIVE PEER REVIEW COMMITTEE MEETING

- Discussion and decision management: Allowing for a productive exchange of ideas that leads to a conclusion

- Action follow-up: Holding individuals accountable for post-meeting assignments so the next meeting will be productive

In case you didn't notice, the first and last elements do not occur during the meeting itself. Thus, half of a successful meeting occurs outside the meeting! Unless there is good preparation and follow-up, meetings will be unproductive.

Before we provide some practical tips on how to accomplish each of these four tasks, let's first look at the role of the committee chair and responsibilities of the committee members to help create a successful meeting.

Role of the Committee Chair

Like the quarterback of a football team, the chair plays the key role in running a meeting. Unfortunately, some chairs assume being the chair gives them the authority to make decisions for the committee. In reality, the chair serves the committee by helping its members make decisions. Here is one way to see that role:

"To be a servant of the group rather than its master ... to assist the group toward the best decision in the most efficient manner possible: to interpret and clarify, move the discussion forward, and bring it to a resolution that everyone understands and accepts as being the will of the meeting, even if individuals do not necessarily agree ... "[1]

This is the concept of servant leadership. The leader sets the example of all the culture values discussed in Chapter 2. For example, if the chair does not follow the procedures for case review discussions designed to reduce bias, then why should the committee members follow it? Just like some quarterbacks ignore the play sent in by the coach and audible at line of scrimmage, some committee chairs deal with situations based on their personal view rather than first checking the playbook.

A critical way the chair serves the committee is in time management. Unfortunately, too many physician leaders walk into a meeting that they chair without any idea what is on the agenda, how long items will take to discuss, or what decisions need to be made. As a committee chair, you have been entrusted to the valuable time of your colleagues. This responsibility may seem most evident during the meeting itself but it begins in the meeting preparation phase and concludes in the follow-up phase. A little extra time spent on your part in preparation and follow-up will yield a tremendous return in savings of the total time spent by your committee. For example, check the care appropriate case reviews and place them on a consent agenda and ensure inquiry letters go out on time so responses are received by the next meeting.

As mentioned earlier, the goal of the meeting is to make decisions. For the chair, this means knowing how to get the committee to make decisions. That is the difference between directive and facilitative decision-making. For example, I have been in peer review committee meetings where the chair presents each case, does most of the talking, and forcefully expresses what he believes is the correct committee decision. Typically silence follows and the decision is not discussed further or even voted on. While this may seem more efficient—Voltaire argued that an enlightened despot is the most efficient form of government—with this directive decision-making approach, eventually the chair will be viewed as overstepping his bounds.

So what is the chair's role in facilitative decision-making? The primary focus is to ensure that conflicting views—if they exist—are encouraged to be expressed and even solicited. The chair needs to know when and how to express his or her own opinion. The "when" is typically after others have been given the opportunity first (i.e., the primary reviewer should present the case). The "how" is for the chair to emphasize that although he or she may have a different point of view, it is the majority view that will stand.

Responsibilities of Committee Members in Meeting Preparation and Management

I am sure you are aware of football teams with a good quarterback but a losing record. Clearly there are other members of the team that have to do their job for the team to succeed. They must all know their role in each play, whether it is blocking, carrying the ball, or receiving a pass. Similarly, in a peer review committee, the committee members must know the playbook of how the committee operates and do their assignments when their number is called.

For example, if the committee rule is to follow the agenda, a member should not intentionally try to redirect discussion to a tangential topic and should respect the chair's request to stay on correct topic. If the policy for case reviews is to complete the review within two weeks, the quality staff should not have to continually request the member complete the review for several additional weeks.

RUNNING AN EFFECTIVE PEER REVIEW COMMITTEE MEETING

How can members meet their responsibilities? First, they should be provided with a clear written outline of the committee policies and procedures and an orientation session with the chair when they join the committee. Incorporating the meeting tips described below into a brief (e.g., one page) document will provide them with a better understanding of how the meeting is run. Second, they need to be open to guidance from the chair and the staff if they misunderstand how the committee works.

Practical Tips for Managing Committee Discussion to Avoid Wasting Physician Time

Here are some effective practices for having productive peer review committee meetings:

- Meeting preparation: Plan your agenda

    - Schedule a routine pre-meeting with the review staff three to five days prior to the meeting to review cases and understand the issues underlying each agenda topic.

    - Hold a pre-meeting with key committee members or invited guests for controversial topics. This is not to determine a backroom pre-meeting decision but air issues in a setting that may create a better understanding and decrease the amount of meeting discussion time.

    - Assign estimated time limits for each agenda item. If the discussion goes longer, let the committee decide if it should be deferred to the next meeting or defer other items.

    - Create a consent agenda. This will have reports or other items not likely to require discussion. However, anyone may ask that an item be moved to the active agenda either for the current meeting (if it is brief) or for next meeting.

- Agenda management

    - Start on time: People will always arrive late unless you establish that you start on time every time.

    - Move the agenda by staying on task and keeping the committee aware when items are exceeding their projected time.

- End on time: People are more likely to commit to a meeting if they know it will not blow up the rest of their schedule. If business is not completed, determine whether some activities between meetings can accelerate the process.

- Discussion and decision management

    - Establish a bias toward constructive input and action at the start of each meeting.

    - Address any potential conflict-of-interest issues before initiating discussion.

    - Solicit active input from all participants and limit the vocal minority.

    - Limit non-productive discussion by politely but firmly reminding the member(s) to focus on the issue at hand.

    - Use skillful interruption to summarize keys points and request feedback.

    - Use the "parking lot" method if tangential or non-agenda issues are raised. This means the member is told, "Great idea, but it is not on the agenda today. Let's put that in the parking lot and we will either come back to it at the end if there is time or place it on the next meeting agenda and research ahead of time for more productive discussion."

    - Suggest a straw vote for determining the level of consensus if points are being repeated.

    - Terminate discussion if it is not progressing toward a decision and assign one or two interested members to research and bring back recommendation.

    - Vote on official items.

- Action follow-up

    - Clarify action items and responsibilities during and at the end of the meeting

    - Have a set meeting with staff for follow-up activities

    - Find out well in advance of the next meeting the status of follow-up items

    - Hold members and staff accountable for persistent lack of follow-up

RUNNING AN EFFECTIVE PEER REVIEW COMMITTEE MEETING

While not all of these practices may be comfortable for your meeting-management style, trying them is the only way you find out if they can make a difference. The key is to be transparent about them so everyone knows the rules. Discussing these practices at your peer review meeting to get buy-in and approval from the committee will help create a culture where the members and the chair are all working from the same playbook.

REFERENCE

1. Jay, Antony. "How to Run a Meeting," *Harvard Business Review* (March, 1976). Accessed 3/1/2013. *http://hbr.org/1976/03/how-to-run-a-meeting/ar/1*

15. Beyond the Hospital Walls: Peer Review in Ambulatory Care and ACOs

Although this book focuses predominately on hospital-based peer review, there is an increasing need to understand how to systematically measure and evaluate physician competency when care is provided outside the hospital or when physicians are accountable to an organization apart from the medical staff. This chapter will address to what extent the systems, methods, and measures of the hospital setting can be translated to other settings and what new approaches may be needed to meet this challenge. However, first let's discuss what is driving this need.

Why Would You Want to Do Peer Review in a Nonhospital Setting?

Evaluating physician ongoing competency outside the hospital is not really new. For example, if a physician is part of a group practice, the group needs to be sure that the physician is competent or the entire group will feel the economic impact. If a freestanding surgicenter desires accreditation, it will need to have a peer review system in place.

However, in a nonregulated environment, it is common for physicians to approach this task in a much looser manner. In the past, practice groups often relied on the hospital credentialing and privileging systems, including peer review, to ensure competency because a significant component of a physician's practice occurred in the hospital. Also, since the data systems and support staff used to support peer review in the hospital setting have significant costs, most groups did the minimal since it was not required. Think of what hospital support for physician performance measurement was like 10 to 20 years ago, before requirements for ongoing professional practice evaluation (OPPE) and core measures raised the bar for peer review support.

So why is today any different? Here are six key factors (there are more) driving the need for creating a more systematic approach to peer review in settings outside the hospital:

CHAPTER 15

1. Rise of the hospitalist: With many primary care physicians abandoning acute care medicine (and hospitalists taking their place), the hospital no longer has the data to ensure these physicians are competent. To avoid the burden of obtaining competency data for these physicians, many medical staffs have created membership categories that do not require hospital privileges. Thus, external groups, like group practices or payers, can no longer use the hospital peer review process as a surrogate for their own.

2. Increase of ambulatory procedures: Over the last decade, many inpatient or hospital facility procedures have moved to the ambulatory settings. Even if these procedures are done in hospital ambulatory facilities with accreditation requirements for peer review, the data systems between the hospital and its ambulatory facility often don't connect.

3. Hospital physician practice acquisition: Hospitals are back in the mode of acquiring physician practices. Last time this occurred in the 1990s and early 2000s, there was less attention paid to obtaining physician quality data because there was quality data available from the medical staff peer review and there was minimal impact on reimbursement. This time, because of reimbursement and malpractice environments, there is greater recognition of the economic risk involved in acquiring physician practices.

4. Medicare EHR requirements for ambulatory care: The Health Information Technology for Economic and Clinical Health Act of 2009 created initial incentives and subsequent penalties for noncompliance for implementing an electronic health record (EHR) that meets the definition of "meaningful use." This applies to all healthcare settings, including ambulatory care. This process is designed to occur over three stages from 2012 to 2016. While the first two stages focused on data capture, sharing, and reporting, the third stage will require improvement in healthcare outcomes.

5. Government and payer incentives and penalties for quality: Both Medicare and commercial payers now link reimbursement to quality data. While this is initially related to acute care, it has progressed to physician reimbursement.

6. Formation of ACOs: With the Patient Protection and Affordable Care Act of 2010, the requirement for physician data has increased, particularly if the physicians choose to participate in an accountable care organization (ACO). Since the ACO approach places the responsibility of physician performance on the physician group in order to benefit from

savings or avoid penalties, to succeed, an ACO will need to implement an ongoing evaluation system to hold physicians accountable (i.e., peer review). Commercial payers are also seeking to reduce costs and increase quality through the ACO approach.

Can You Do Peer Review in the Nonhospital Setting?

All of these factors imply that physician performance needs to be evaluated and, if necessary, improved in the nonhospital setting. This raises two questions:

1. Should (and will) this still be done by physicians?

2. Do the hospital medical staff methods for peer review still apply?

The first question is based on whether the organizations accountable for physician performance, either employers or contractors, still hold to the belief that physicians need to be involved in determining the competency of their colleagues. If not, physician performance measurement could be done by nonphysician managers as an administrative process based on performance data, like any other employee. However, most organizations, particularly those that are physician-owned or -led, believe that some form of peer review process, where physicians hold each other accountable, is still important. The remainder of the discussion in this chapter is based on that premise.

The second question essentially asks: Without the regulatory requirements of a self-governing medical staff, even though the evaluation is performed by physicians, does it need to look the same as a hospital-based method? Based on my observation of the range of approaches already in place in these settings, that answer is a qualified, "No." While it is likely that some basic elements of the medical staff system should be retained and that the culture goal of physician improvement should be the same, compared to the medical staff model, the structure and processes certainly may vary and, in some cases, for the better. The 10 steps described in Chapter 11 are generally applicable to how your organization should approach this challenge. The remainder of this chapter addresses how peer review can be accomplished in this brave new world.

What Data Can You Obtain From the Hospital and What Are You Willing to Share?

Most new ideas are built on previous ones. Similarly, if you are trying to build a data-based peer review system, it is more efficient to start by determining whether you can obtain data that is already being collected on physician competency. Obviously, for inpatient data that would be from the hospital. However, this is not the same as the past practice of relying on the hospital's credentialing and peer review decisions mentioned earlier. Real peer review in the nonhospital setting means obtaining the actual data and evaluating it in your own setting.

For example, you may wish the hospital to inform your group practice when an adverse patient outcome occurs that involved a physician from your group. Then your group's peer review process would have access to the inpatient medical record and determine whether there was an improvement opportunity based on your group's standards and expectations of its physicians. Another example is that you may wish to obtain OPPE data for your physicians and evaluate it using your group's targets for excellent and acceptable performance.

On the other hand, the hospital has physicians on its staff for which it has no data because they practice solely in an ambulatory setting. If they maintain privileges, there is a need for OPPE data. Even if they do not have specific privileges at the hospital, their membership on the medical staff implies to the patients that the hospital has some understanding that they are quality physicians. Thus, the hospital's reputation is potentially at stake. So the hospital, in a quid pro quo for providing your group with inpatient data, would like to get data from your group practice on Healthcare Effectiveness Data and Information Set (HEDIS) measures for ambulatory care.

Sounds simple, doesn't it? Unfortunately, it may not be depending on your state's statutes for peer review protection, fairness issues related to your hospital's medical staff composition, and political issues related to physician groups' relationships with the hospital. First, let's start with the legal issues.

In order for you to receive data from the hospital and not have any effect on the hospital medical staff's protection from discoverability, you need a sharing agreement that meets your state's requirements. In some states, like California, a group practice can be designated as a recognized entity for quality and peer review protection if the group has certain policies and procedures in place. As such, the group can receive data from other entities like a hospital under a data-sharing agreement and maintain protection for both organizations. Other states are more restrictive on data sharing. Before you contemplate any data-sharing agreement, you should consult your legal counsel as to what is allowable in your state.

The issue of fairness arises if the hospital desires data from your physician group in exchange for the data it provides. Even though a two-way street approach for data may seem the most fair, ironically it may be more unfair to the physicians in your group if the data is used by the medical staff for peer review and credentialing. If the medical staff is composed of a number of physician groups and solo practitioners and similar data are not available from them, the physicians in your group may feel they are being held unfairly to a higher standard. This data double standard would be true even if the ambulatory care physicians were employed by the hospital. Thus, unless the medical staff determines that all physicians, regardless of their group affiliation or employment status, would submit the same data, it is best to keep this as a one-way data flow from the hospital to the practice group.

The political issues related to physician groups' relationships with the hospital may arise from the hospital administration's concerns. If a physician group is perceived as desiring to use shared adverse-event data to try to interfere with the hospital performance improvement or risk management processes, then the hospital is less willing to share this information. For example, if an adverse event resulted in a case for peer review, in a sharing agreement, the physician group would be made aware of the event and could review the record and talk to the shared physician. However, if the group wanted to interview other caregivers involved in the event, such as the nurses or other hospital employees, that might be beyond the bounds of what the hospital would allow. These types of issues should be resolved while developing a solid sharing agreement.

Peer Review Outside the Hospital: How Should You Organize It?

Whether you are trying to understand the quality care provided solely by ambulatory care physicians or the totality of care provided by physicians participating in a group practice or ACO, the three questions regarding peer review to address are: how to structure it, what data to obtain, and who will get it.

This chapter is not intended to provide a complete discussion of all the options for all possible practice settings. Rather, it will focus on some of the peer review structure options to consider for three of the most common settings where this issue is being raised: hospital-employed primary care physician practices, independent multi-specialty physician group practices (with or without hospitalists), and ACOs.

Hospital-employed primary care physician practice

As a hospital builds its primary care base, typically these physicians represent a mixture of those who were recruited directly by the hospital and those who were incorporated into the group by practice acquisition. In the case of recruitment, while there is typically a defined administrative structure in place, there is often no medical quality evaluation structure. Physicians are assigned to clinics and there is often a medical director for the practice, but the responsibility and structure for managing physician quality is often ill-defined. Because the physicians are hospital employees and typically medical staff members, the hospital often assumes that the medical staff will fulfill that role. Thus peer review can be organized as if the group was an independant group practice.

When practices are acquired, particularly small practices, it can be even more challenging because the physicians are used to a practice culture where they operated with relative autonomy. While a practice acquisition expansion may undergo financial performance due diligence, it is not uncommon that a quality due diligence, aside from pending malpractice litigations, is not performed. Since these practices usually have minimal internal quality evaluation systems and the physicians are often already medical staff members, again the hospital assumes that the medical staff will take on the responsibility of quality oversight.

So what are the options for oversight and evaluation of physician quality for hospital-owned primary care practices? Below are two approaches to consider.

Formally integrate this responsibility into the medical staff peer review structure

If the medical staff has a single multi-specialty committee, then the primary care practice information would flow to that committee. If the medical staff has department-based peer review, the relevant department committee would be responsible. Alternately, the medical staff can create a department of primary care (or a section within an existing department) and that chair would be responsible.

How would the primary care physicians be evaluated under this structure? Unusual events and issues regarding outpatient care that result in serious outcomes, with or without hospitalization, would be evaluated by case review. Rate and rule data would be evaluated by the relevant medical staff department chair using OPPE reports.

The advantages of this structure are that no sharing agreement would be needed and you would not have to create a new peer review structure. The disadvantages are that the medical staff may be hesitant to take on this responsibility, it may create fairness issues relative to non-employed physicians (as discussed earlier), and the data support process would typically fall to the existing peer review staff, who aren't as knowledgeable about ambulatory care so they give it a lower priority than the hospital-based peer review activities. This will most likely be the case unless dedicated staff is added to take on this responsibility.

Create a separate primary care group practice peer review structure

Since the physicians do not practice in the hospital, they do not need hospital privileges and can be evaluated qualitatively by the hospital as a low- or no-volume physician. Thus, peer review can be organized as if the group was an independent practice group. The options for structuring this approach will be discussed in the section on independent group practice model.

The main advantage of the primary care group practice peer review structure approach is that you are no longer constrained by the hospital's medical staff politics and structures. This will also force you to seriously think about the approach to physician performance improvement in the context of the group's desired culture. Another advantage is that this approach also covers physicians in the group who practice at more distant locations and do not need to be members of your hospital's medical staff.

The main disadvantage of this approach is the need to have a separate quality support infrastructure. However, it will help better define the resources needed and make sure the group is the priority. Physician quality measurement should be a cost of doing business in today's environment and should be factored into the budget rather than an afterthought. Because the group is owned by the hospital, for accreditation purposes the information must somehow flow to the hospital board. This can be done either directly to the board like all other employees to avoid medical staff political engagement with the group or through the medical executive committee.

Independent multi-specialty physician group practice

A multi-specialty group practice in many ways may look like a hospital medical staff with the diversity of specialties involved and the tendency to assume that each specialty should be responsible for its own area. However, the group practice may often have a culture that is distinctly different from the medical staff because it can define its own culture. It may be ahead of the medical staff in terms of its focus on physician improvement or it may have a more business-like performance-driven culture.

Whatever the culture, unlike most medical staffs, leadership is typically appointed rather than elected (i.e., a medical director for either a specialty or a facility) and paid to perform the oversight of quality in some manner as part of its job description. However, in speaking with group practice medical directors over the years, I have found that the authority given to manage quality is generally not concomitant with the responsibilities assigned to them. Sometimes the quality medical director is different from the administrative medical director so there may be a disassociation between quality performance issues and other aspects (e.g., productivity of the physician's performance).

Many groups have a medical staff model for corrective action where a physician dismissal requires action by the entire board. In one large group practice clinic, of the approximately 500 physician members, every physician was a board member except for a few physicians who had recently joined the clinic.

The main difference between the multi-specialty group practice and the hospital-owned primary care group is that the multi-specialty practice needs to be concerned about the care provided by its physicians in all patient care settings. Thus, it needs information from both the hospital on the inpatient care provided by its physicians as well as from its own clinics or offices. As discussed earlier in this chapter, it will need some type of sharing agreement to fully evaluate its physicians. But the structure defining who evaluates that information and the functions that it performs have the same options that are available to a medical staff, which were discussed in Chapter 4: specialty medical director, specialty committee, or multi-specialty committee.

The key question the group needs to address is whether the perception of bias will affect the group's culture. I have found that in speaking with physicians who work in a group practice setting, physician satisfaction within the group, in addition to income, is still based on the sense of fairness in the evaluation process and the feeling that they are part of a high-quality team. Thus, peer review models that address these issues will be more successful. On the other hand, with strong physician leadership, and a culture focused on team performance and clear performance expectations, medical groups may be able to use a more direct approach for performance evaluation.

The medical director model is most susceptible to personal bias. The specialty committee is susceptible to specialty bias and may not be able to drive improvement. Similar to the hospital medical staff, the least biased approach would be through a multi-specialty committee. If the group has multiple large facilities that are geographically dispersed, it may even wish to have a local multi-specialty committee at each setting with a central oversight committee.

What then is the role of the medical director? Typically, it would be similar to the functions of a department chair, by obtaining and evaluating aggregate data like in OPPE and working with the physicians on improvement opportunities. If the medical director also has administrative authority, she or he would make recommendations regarding a physician's membership or privileges to either an appropriate committee or through a management structure.

Should the medical directors comprise the multi-specialty committee, or should the membership come from those without administrative roles? The answer would be based on the group practice's culture and goals regarding physician engagement. If the group desires greater engagement, the committee should certainly include, either in whole or in part, physicians who are not in an administrative role.

In terms of quality support infrastructure, in the past, many groups did not have this in place. The recognition that this infrastructure is a cost of doing business in the current reimbursement environment should be a motivating factor to determine what the resources are needed to get the job done well. A single multi-specialty committee performing its role in measurement system management can help guide this process.

Accountable care organizations

Unlike the medical staff or the group practice setting, the ACO is usually starting from scratch so there is typically no structure in place. Like the multi-specialty group practice, the ACO needs to assess physician performance in all care settings. However, because an ACO will often include physicians who are employed as well as those in private practice groups of varying sizes (including solo practitioners), the cultural challenges are more pronounced. The issues of fairness and bias will be accentuated compared to the single group practice setting. Although the physicians participating in the ACO will often not be a direct duplication of the medical staff, many of the cultural characteristics of the medical staff will affect the ACO culture, for good or for ill. Thus, the ACO leadership will need to determine how the medical staff peer review culture will affect the new organization and what it needs to do either to reinforce it, or, more likely, to change it.

One of most important cultural characteristics for ACOs to address is creating physician accountability at a much higher level than the typical medical staff is willing to impose. The economic viability of the ACO depends on it. In this more structured practice environment, the peer review process will need to have a greater emphasis on rapid change of physician practice. With that in mind, let's look at some options for an ACO peer review structure.

Again, like the multi-specialty group, the three approaches (i.e., specialty medical director, specialty committee, or multi-specialty committee) are available to the ACO. The question is which approach is more likely to exert influence required to change physician practice. This influence will include monetary incentives or penalties that are intertwined with clinical performance.

There appear to be two needs driving the approach to influence. Because care in an ACO needs to be coordinated, a multi-specialty structure would be best suited to evaluate these issues. However, because of the need for rapid influence, some form of specialty involvement will probably be needed since specialty-specific practice patterns will need to be modified. Defining specialty medical directors who would serve the function of the department chairs would accomplish this role. These medical directors could also comprise the membership of the multi-specialty committee which would increase the rapid deployment and accountability of the medical directors. However, unlike the medical staff department chair who is often elected by physicians in his or her specialty, it is more likely that the medical director in an ACO will be appointed by the ACO board. Therefore, to increase physician engagement, the ACO may wish to also have nonmedical directors as well on the committee.

Peer Review Outside the Hospital: What Can You Measure?

For any of the above settings, the measurement challenge has three components:

1. The measurement framework and expectations you will set

2. The data sources you will use

3. The resources that you have to obtain the data and support the process

These challenges will be viewed based on how they compare to the same issues for medical staff peer review discussed in previous chapters.

The measurement frameworks and expectations were discussed in Chapter 7. The core competencies framework certainly is applicable to any of these settings. If the physicians are members of a medical staff that already use that framework, it would resonate better with them than adopting a new one. The one measurement area that is different from the hospital medical staff compared to the other settings is productivity. There are two options I have seen for this issue:

1. Include productivity measures within the peer review structure under the core competency of systems-based practice

2. Address productivity administratively apart from peer review

The key is to review your competency framework to make sure you consider obtaining data for all competencies relevant to the ambulatory care setting.

The data source issue begins with what you can obtain from the hospital via a sharing agreement discussed earlier and what you can obtain from the ambulatory care setting that would provide a complete picture of a physician's performance. Since the options are the same regardless of whether the entity is an employed ambulatory care group, independent group practice, or ACO, for purposes of this discussion, I will refer to any of these as the "organization." The purpose of this chapter is to provide guidelines on what types of measure are useful and how to select them rather than providing a specific indicator list. Let's look at the types of data and resources needed for the three types of indicators (i.e., review, rules, and rates) and see how they would be applied in these organizational settings.

Case review

The presumption in the ambulatory care setting is that fewer issues would rise to the level of severity requiring detailed case review like those in the acute care setting. However, if the organization is concerned about the total care provided by its practitioners, it needs to review the acute care events as well to identify improvement opportunities. In addition, there are some issues detected in the ambulatory care that would warrant the case review approach, such as an office-based procedure, signifcant complication, missed diagnosis, or misdiagnosis resulting in patient harm. Thus, the organization's peer review committee needs to define a set of review indicators with inclusion and exclusion criteria to ensure fairness in case selection that address both the acute and ambulatory care settings, and then apply a similar approach to the case review process described in Chapter 6.

How can you identify these cases? At a minimum, a sharing agreement should allow the hospital to make the organization aware of the event and provide access to the medical record. If the organization and the hospital have an integrated EHR, this is much easier. The organization could then review the case in its own peer review process and determine improvement opportunities. Whether the hospital shares its own peer review findings and improvement efforts depends on the extent of the sharing agreement and how closely tied the organization is to the hospital.

In addition to the hospital identifying events for review, once the peer review committee selects its ambulatory case review indicators, it needs to establish a mechanism to identify these cases. Typically this will come from referrals from clinic staff and patient complaints. However, if the ambulatory care EHR can be mined to identify such events, it will increase the effectiveness of the case identification.

One area of confusion regarding case review that comes up particularly in the ambulatory care setting is the process of medical directors reviewing randomly selected charts for specific (e.g., was the Hgb A1C ordered?) or general (e.g., did the visit note acknowledge abnormal lab values?) issues. This is actually an audit rather than true case review as the term is used in this book. Here, the medical director is acting as a data collector (and an expensive one) often aggregating the findings into a rule or rate approach. Whether this process is useful compared to the time and expense relative to the organizational benefit is an individual organizational decision. However, to the greatest extent possible, such audits can be done by nonphysician resources based on clear criteria (e.g., core measures) with the medical director receiving the data like other rule or rate measures.

Rule and rate indicators

As discussed in Chapter 5, rule indicators typically measure compliance with defined practices (e.g., ordering the recommended antibiotic) or policies (e.g., hand washing) that could be improved by timely feedback for self-improvement for individual occurrences and targets to identify patterns over a defined time period. Rate indicators typically measure processes or outcomes that have reasonable frequencies of occurrence and where feedback can occur for the aggregate data at specific time intervals.

Inpatient physician rule and rate indicators may already be measured by the medical staff and reported via OPPE. Thus, a hospital sharing agreement should provide the organization access to the semiannual OPPE reports for its physicians that have inpatient activity. If the hospital has invested in data systems for OPPE data, this will provide a good start. If not, you should encourage the hospital to do so, especially if you are an ACO. Either way your committee's primary focus will be on the ambulatory care setting.

Whether you determine to use rule or rate indicators for a given issue can vary by the organization. The questions for organizations outside the hospital are: first, what should you measure and then what type, rule or rate, would work best based on volume and data collection resources. Just as with review indicators, the peer review committee needs to determine what ambulatory care practices are important enough to evaluate by rule or rate measures, which form of feedback is best, and how it will obtain the data. Here are some places to find data and how to relate them to the six core competencies:

- Data already being collected and submitted electronically such as HEDIS or physician quality reporting system (PQRS) measures. Many of these measures would fall under the core competency of medical knowledge. Although these may be treated as a rate indicator, they are often useful as a rule indicator if compliance is generally high and feedback is desired on an individual event basis to get to 100% compliance goals. As the pressure on meaningful use compliance increases, this data should be obtainable by queries of your EHR instead of manual data abstraction.

- Abstract patient records for general care measures or for policies specific to your organization's functions. These measures typically fall under the core competency of interpersonal and communication skills or systems-based practice. For example, abstracting random charts to ensure key elements of care are addressed in a patient visit could be useful for primary care internists as a measure of communication within the team. If this is done manually by physicians, making the cost high, use a relatively small sample and treat it as a rule indicator so feedback is reviewed on single instances of noncompliance. To the extent this can be done by nonphysician abstractors or through EHR queries, the cost can be reduced and the sample size increased. A second example might be for referral patterns that may reflect over- or under-utilization of consultants as a measure of systems-based practice in the use of resources. That information should be obtainable from the billing system based on coding data.

- Patient perception data either from complaints or patient satisfaction surveys. The questions patients are asked typically relate to interpersonal skills. Since the encounters in the ambulatory care setting tend to be with individual physicians, the survey attribution for survey data tends to be much better than in the hospital setting.

- Specialty societies or specialty boards are another data source. In some specialties, physicians participating in ongoing Maintenance of Certification regularly submit data to their medical specialty board. If the organization found it useful, it could either request the information from the physicians if all are participating or determine to collect the data internally from physicians. These measures typically fall under medical knowledge.

- Patient access is a key issue in ambulatory care. Measures related to cancelled clinics or appointment availability may reflect either professionalism or systems-based practice. This information should be obtained through the patient scheduling system for integrated groups. This may be more difficult for ACOs unless a scheduling infrastructure is in place.

Ultimately, in the ambulatory setting today, what you measure will be affected by your organization's willingness to invest in the resources needed to understand and manage quality as an essential part of your business rather than as a regulatory requirement.

16 Creating Effective Peer Review Policies and Procedures

I hope this book has provided useful concepts and practical approaches that will help you and your fellow medical staff leaders take your peer review programs to the next level. You may need to tweak only a few aspects of your program, but others may need to make fairly substantial changes. For the latter group, the transformation necessary may seem overwhelming, so this chapter lays out a general work plan for redesigning your peer review program using the concepts discussed in this book.

What Do Your Policies and Procedures Need to Cover?

Too often policies for peer review are written to make the accrediting body happy rather than to truly guide your peer review program. They are often vague in regard to what is actually done. Your policies and procedures should describe how your program is designed to work. Using this book as a guide, the following elements make for a good set of documents to support your peer review program.

Purpose and goals: A statement of what you are trying to achieve by conducting peer review from an operational, cultural, and regulatory perspective in the manner described by your policies.

Definitions of key terms including:

- Peer review

- Ongoing professional practice evaluation (OPPE)

- Focused professional practice evaluation (FPPE)

- Peer review body

- Peer

- Peer review data sources

Effective Peer Review, Third Edition

- Practitioner competencies framework

- Conflict of interest

Structure: A detailed charter describing the committee(s) conducting peer review including:

- Peer review quality, cultural, and regulatory goals

- Responsibilities

- Membership

- Oversight and reporting

Peer review procedures

- **Information management:** The methods to ensure information is handled appropriately

- **Confidentiality:** How and where written documents and electronic records will be maintained, who will have access, and how long they will be retained

- **Use:** How information will be used for performance improvement and credentialing

- **Internal peer review:** Descriptions of the circumstances, participants, procedures, and indicators for case review, OPPE, and FPPE related to OPPE including:

  – Selection process for measures for case review and OPPE

  – A list of all measures designated as either review, rule, or rates with targets for FPPE and physician attribution for the rule and rate measures

  – Procedures for case review including the case rating form

  – Process for indicator data evaluation for OPPE

  – Procedure for conducting FPPE based on OPPE issues

- **External peer review:** Description of the circumstances, authorization, use of the report, and practitioner involvement

These documents can be in a single policy or may be organized into an overall policy with more detailed procedures or lists provided as attachments.

Redesigning Your Peer Review Program: A Step-by-Step Guide

For those pursuing a significant redesign of your peer review program, this will take both thoughtfulness and physician leadership time. Having worked with medical staffs on this process over the past 12 years, I find that success for this endeavor requires a well-thought-out plan and the energy and persistence to complete it, whether you do this with the assistance of an external consultant or use internal leadership resources.

What follows is a work plan that is described as a series of 10 steps. Some medical staffs will need to spend more time on some steps compared to other medical staffs depending on their degree of consensus and expertise. While the order, in general, will be the same for most organizations, you may be able to start some steps before you complete others.

Step 1: Confirm the medical staff leaders' ownership in the peer review process

Unless the medical staff leaders recognize that this is their responsibility, not just a way to comply with regulatory and accreditation requirements, any changes may be doomed to failure. The earlier chapters of this book should provide you with the background necessary for this discussion. Another option is to send the leaders to outside educational programs where they can learn from other physicians.

Step 2: Commission a design group and create a work plan

This work is complex and requires input from current and past leaders. Rather than assign it to an existing committee, create a special work group and give them a work plan. Using the concepts discussed in this book and these 10 steps, you can identify the key tasks or deliverables for the design group and the estimated time for the start and completion of each task. Then use the work plan at each meeting to monitor progress.

Step 3: Adopt a philosophy and framework of peer review that will define your culture

Before getting into the details of the process, decide how you wish to approach peer review and which dimensions of physician performance to address. Then develop the expectations that will drive your physician performance improvement program.

CHAPTER 16

Step 4: Benchmark with others

Don't reinvent the wheel. Look at what others do, compare it to what you do, and decide whether that would work for you. You can also benchmark by looking at other individual organizations, reviewing available literature, attending conferences, networking, or using consultants for on-site education or facilitating the project. In fact, this book is a benchmarking source.

Step 5: Define the peer review structure that meets your culture goals

This critical decision requires thoughtful discussion. Discuss whether the current peer review structure can be modified or whether it would be better to blow it up and create it anew. Weigh the pros and cons for each of the current approaches described in Chapter 4. Narrow the options to those that are most realistic given your medical staff organization, and select the best one. Then draft a charter that describes it.

Step 6: Define the case review process

This has two components: the procedure for performing reviews and the case rating system. Chapter 6 provides some options for both components. Then embody your choices in a draft case rating form that is easy to use and pilot-test it. You can even test the draft tool using the current committee structure. Committees often waste time trying to make something perfect only to find that, once they try it, it needs to be modified.

Step 7: Develop policies and procedures that describe your peer review structure and process

The basic documents needed for a good peer review program are described in the beginning of this chapter. These documents should be easy to understand and should not be written in "bylaws language." If you are accredited by The Joint Commission, be sure that the terms ongoing professional practice evaluation (OPPE) and focused professional practice evaluation (FPPE), as well as the general competencies, are reflected in these documents, along with the processes to implement them.

Step 8: Develop efficient and reliable performance measures

Chapters 5, 7, and 8 provide a guide to creating the right types of measures. Start by cataloguing your current measures, and then discuss them. Then determine which of these measures will be part of the OPPE report. At this stage, the design group should decide if it will work on the OPPE and feedback reports or have that task be handled by a different group, such as the credentials committee or the new committee structure.

CREATING EFFECTIVE PEER REVIEW POLICIES AND PROCEDURES

Step 9: Obtain feedback, modify accordingly, and submit for approval

You can do this with the design group work products at each step or at the end. Getting feedback early is preferable, as it can prevent the design group from getting locked into a concept. Typically, feedback is first obtained from the medical executive committee (MEC) and then from the medical staff and the departments. The MEC should ultimately approve all documents, but whether approval by the medical staff is necessary depends on your medical staff bylaws.

Step 10: Orient and train physicians in the new system

Create a training session to explain the new system and tools to all members of the peer review committee. It can also be useful to create a manual that includes all the aforementioned documents and appropriate background materials. Each committee member should be given a copy. The manual can then be consulted at committee meetings, and if there is a question about how to proceed, everyone can refer to the appropriate policy.

Should You Do This Yourself or Get Some Help?

As a speaker and author who provides education and training to physician leaders to help them take on a project of this magnitude on their own, and as a consultant that works directly with medical staff design groups, I have seen that both approaches can work. The choice may be based on the organization's philosophy on the use of consultants, the medical staff's openness to "outsiders" telling them what to do, the availability of internal or healthcare system expertise, or financial constraints. Since consultants will cost money, why would you want to hire one?

The two main reasons for using a consultant for a project of this type are time and customization. A good consultant should ultimately save you time in four ways by:

1. Providing ideas and documents that will expedite your choices

2. Facilitating the design group sessions to ensure they are productive

3. Managing the project to move it forward to implementation

4. Increasing the medical staff buy-in to drive the culture change promoted by the new system

CHAPTER 16

A good consultant should also help you make wise choices that reflect your organization and not just provide turnkey approaches that may not work in your organization. This implies that if you do choose to use a consultant either for an entire project or for parts of it, make sure his or her philosophy and approach to peer review matches your medical staff goals and desired culture.

The issue is not whether a chief medical officer or chief of staff is smart enough to do these things; it is whether he or she is knowledgeable enough and has sufficient time and political capital to spend. Just this past year, I worked on several projects with medical staff leaders who were initially charged with doing this internally. After the projects were completed, each told me how much time the medical staff had wasted at numerous meetings prior to getting help and that they wished they had gotten assistance a year earlier. Given the true cost of physician meeting time discussed in Chapter 14, they saw the cost of consulting assistance as a bargain.

I have also worked with organizations that do have the capabilities and time to do the design work on their own (often using this book as a guide) and then ask for assistance for training and implementation. While I often found that not all of the pieces were in place or some choices were made that might have impacts that were not considered, with a little additional help, a solid program could be initiated.

My personal goal over the past 12 years of my career has been to assist medical staffs to create the kind of peer review program that helps physicians improve patient care in a culture that allows them to learn and grow. Whether I have the opportunity to do this through books or by working with you personally, the reason I enjoy what I do is that I have learned that there are many physician leaders who want to do this well and, with a little help, can make a real difference for the patients and physicians in their community. I know that I am blessed to have the privilege to work alongside them in this effort.